THE
HAPPY BODY

MASTERING *EXERCISE* CHOICES

ALSO BY JERZY GREGOREK

Non-Fiction
The Happy Body (2009)
The Happy Body Mind (forthcoming)

Poetry
Sacred and Scared (2014)
A Healthy Mirror for Change (2014)
Family Tree (2015)

Dialogues
The Happy Body: Mastering Food Choices (2015)
The Happy Body: Mastering Rest Choices (2015)

Translations (with Aniela Gregorek)
Late Confession by Józef Baran (1997)
Watermarks by Bogusław Żurakowski 2000)
Her Miniature by Zbigniew Czuchajowski (2000)
In a Flash by Józef Baran (2000)
The Poetry of Maurycy Szymel (2004)
The Shy Hand of a Jew by Maurycy (Mosze) Szymel (2013)
Native Foreigners (2015)

Videos
The Happy Body Ambience (2013)
The Happy Body Exercise Program (2014)

THE
HAPPY BODY
MASTERING *EXERCISE* CHOICES

Dialogues by
Jerzy Gregorek

The Happy Body Press
Woodside, California
2015

Easy choices, difficult life.
Difficult choices, easy life.

Please direct inquiries to:

The Happy Body Press
104 Alta Mesa Rd.
Woodside, CA 94062
E-mail: thbp@thehappybody.com

ISBN 9780996243933

First Edition

The Happy Body: Mastering Exercise Choices
by Jerzy Gregorek

Cover image, "The Master Chooses," by Jerzy Gregorek

Cover and text design by Alexander Atkins Design, Inc.

Manufactured and printed in the US, on acid-free paper.

To my clients, who made me conscious of the struggle between the Fatalist and the Master, and the resulting inner dialogues

CONTENTS

PROLOGUE

Exercise has the power to make you better, whether you need more energy because you are too tired during the day, you need to restore your health after an illness or a major injury, or you want to become a world champion. In the past, we knew that exercise gave you these qualities, but we also knew that it required strategy and technique aimed at specific goals, usually with the help of knowledgeable trainers and coaches, always with self-evaluation and a commitment to progress. When strategies were not working to move one forward to the desired goal, there was a realization that something had to be done differently or better.

But that power of exercise was lost in the early 90's.

In 1988, when I worked as a personal trainer at Gold's Gym in North Hollywood, where more than a thousand people trained daily, mostly using free weights, there were four pieces of cardiovascular equipment – two treadmills and two lifecycles. Their main purpose was for 10-minute warm-ups before a workout. Most people had personal trainers, or had them at least while learning basic skills. The purpose of exercising in the gym was to get stronger, more flexible, and faster. If people wanted to lose weight, they knew that exercise was not the solution. For them it was obvious that the only option for losing weight was eating less. It would not have occurred to them that the answer was getting on the treadmill.

But as Americans got heavier and more obsessed with losing weight, exercise machines started to fill the gyms. The number of lifecycles and treadmills doubled every year. One day, a new lifecycle arrived with a digital display that provided a minute-by-minute readout of calories burned. People loved the idea of knowing how many calories they burned — of watching the calories add up on the display — and they began to spend more time on machines and less on training in the gym.

People started competing to see who could burn the most calories in an hour or in a day. Records circulated in the gym, inspiring others to break them. But gradually, people stopped caring about breaking records and started just enjoying the ride. Over time, as the challenges were removed, walking on a treadmill for 30 or 60 minutes became boring so people began reading books, listening to music, or watching movies using personal laptops. The machine manufacturers made new designs that would allow a person to watch a movie or the news or listen to any piece of music. People were on autopilot, discon- nected from exercise as a purpose.

Becoming stronger or more flexible became unimportant and growing muscle became irrelevant. We became obsessed with counting calories, and whatever could help us to burn more we would try – super foods, high intensity routines claiming to burn hundreds calories in minutes, special supplements coming from other continents, even drinking more water.

To our surprise, in spite of all our efforts to lose weight, we became weaker and more obese. After all the programs we tried, not being able to accept responsibility for our misfortune, we began blaming the food industry and fat genes. Even worse, we lost the culture of training with focus on improvement.

What was really happening to us?

When we were little and did not know that two plus two was four, we struggled to understand it, and our teachers and parents worked hard to help us. As soon as we comprehended the answer we entertained everyone with our knowledge. We enjoyed it when they reacted with applause and smiles. We liked the fact that doing the math had become easy. But our happiness did not last long because soon we were asked more difficult questions – what is two plus three, and after that, three plus three. Our education became one of constantly acquiring new knowledge and solving more difficult puzzles, with fewer moments of entertainment when we showed off our knowledge. The more difficult learning became, the more we wanted entertainment and the more we disliked education. Slowly, we removed education from our lives and replaced it with entertainment. We stopped accepting new challenges and forgot the idea of constantly seeking improvement.

Because of progress in medicine, we live longer than ever. More and more, medicine provides interventions that help us when we are sick. Getting the right pills when we become ill can be life saving. Surgery on a broken leg can save a person from limping forever and therefore having lower the quality of life. Here the body is healed and returns to a previous condition. If, however, we have high cholesterol or high blood pressure and we take medicine for it, the medicine helps us to control the condition, but never to heal it to the point where we can stop using pills. We become dependent on these medicines, with all their side effects and potential to cause other health problems. We choose the easy path, even though it does not give us a solution.

But we know the solution to all health-related conditions is in lifestyle. If we want to lower our cholesterol, we need to change our eating and exercise habits. It means we need to be able to do what is good for us although we do not like it. It means we need to stop repeating two plus two is four and start seeking the answer to what is two plus three, three plus three, and so on. Otherwise, we can't change the path we are on.

Aniela's father had diabetes when he was in his early 60s, and he would not stop eating chicken skin, even though his doctor told him he would die if he continued. He simply said, "Life without eating chicken skin is not worth living." For him, two plus three was too difficult. He preferred eating what he did not need and, by doing so, to leave his family, who desperately needed him. He did not hear their voices—they were drowned out by his own *fatalistic voice*, which eventually caused him to lose his leg, and shortly after, his life.

Change for the better happens when education

happens. This means we need to regain the desire for education that enables us to do what we were never able to do before. Day by day, we make what is difficult easy and in that way we become stronger, more flexible, and healthier.

What stops us?

There is a powerful voice in all of us, at times, that embodies that fatalistic attitude. The Fatalist in us does anything to ensure that we fail. This voice will say, for example: "You are too old," "It is impossible," "It's too hard" – the Fatalist will say anything to stop us from getting better. At the same time, there is another voice, the Master, that has the ability to assert control over our actions, to do what we believe is right, even when it's hard. But the Master gets tired, its job is more difficult, and the Fatalist is always there to offer easy entertainment, a distraction from the more difficult task of taking the next step forward.

We need to learn that change only comes from confronting what is difficult and believing that what is difficult can be mastered over time. Just as two plus two once seemed difficult when we were children, overcoming the Fatalist in us will also get easier if we seek the education we need. It's easy to believe that pills can fix what our lifestyle has created, that we are doing enough if we are ticking away calories on the treadmill while watching a movie.

We want to be strong and healthy, but when the Fatalist in us is stronger than the Master, it becomes impossible. With adequate practice, however, this can all be changed. We are all able to awaken inside of us the voice of the Master and realize what we would never had thought was possible.

A Plea to the Medical Community

You are the best thing that has ever happened to us. You have found cures for many diseases that previously killed millions. You have showed us the importance of better hygiene. For a century, we have gone to see you whenever we needed to deliver a baby, recover from sickness or simply felt weak and wanted to understand why. Every time, you served us with your devotion, knowledge and contemporary scientific medicine, to help us with our illnesses and conditions that worsen our health.

Having written poetry for more than thirty years, I have learned that the most difficult and moving art is to write about unfortunate people. Writing glorious poems about how great we are is easy but writing poems about how shameful or destructive we are is difficult. It calls for great courage and humility to share moments that have made our lives worse, in order that they can be felt but not repeated.

Humankind today is in an unfortunate situation. Life today is not asking you anymore to be a scientist. It is asking you to be an artist. Our health does not get worse because we are sick or we get older. Today we become

obese and develop conditions related to overeating—
high blood pressure, osteoporosis, type II diabetes and
others—which could easily be prevented.

We want you to keep searching for new drugs to help
us with all our ailments and maybe one day to extend our
lifespans even further than today. But until these drugs
are available, we ask that you inspire us to eat consciously
and to create for ourselves the internal drive to listen and
follow the voice of the Master within us. Often you tell
us to lose weight or exercise but observing you with the
same unhealthy conditions discourages us, causing us to
lose our struggle to achieve a healthy body weight.

We turn again to you for help. We know that it will
be difficult for you to become more than you are but we
do not know where else to turn. You are the vital pillar
that must support our health. You have the potential to
change our situations for the better and we hope that you
will live up to the task.

NOT ONLY

The doctor told his patient,
"You are diabetic.
Don't wait any longer—lose weight."
"What about you?
You're obese, too."
The doctor did not say anything
but he could not stop thinking about it.
Later, he shared the story with his colleague

who told him, "I thought
you had noticed that the doctor's
calling has changed."
"So it isn't just saving lives anymore?"
"Not only that. It's even bigger.
We've become medicine itself."
"But how can a doctor heal?"
"He climbs the tallest mountain."
"But I wasn't taught that.
It's not my responsibility."
"What is,
if not
becoming healing?"

INTRODUCTION
Costly Failures, Precious Miracles

There are times in life when we feel overwhelmed and nothing seems to work. Whatever we plan requires weeks or months to achieve and we do not feel as if we have that much time. The sense of urgency in us is heightened. The thought that we need to fix the problem tells us that immediate results are needed. Planning to actually achieve the desired results becomes impossible. We begin to worry and become anxious about our future. The pursuit of anything ends up as failure. We blame our misfortune on our parents, friends, God—whomever comes to mind. We want to go to sleep but we do not want to wake up.

When this feeling dominates our life, it is impossible for us to recover on our own. We need help and we are lucky when the right person appears at the right time in our life and has time to drag us off our deathbed. At such times, people who love us check us into rehab centers or similar places where we can recover in ourselves the desire to care about our life.

During my 30 years of practice, I have worked with thousands of people, about five percent of whom were in this impossible stage. They did not come to me on their own. Usually they were sent by spouses, parents or friends. When I asked them why they came, the answers were: my wife sent me, my brother sent me, my mother sent me and so on. Sometimes it was a 16-year-old boy, sometimes a 40-year-old woman or a 60-year-old man.

Despite the differences in age, there was one common belief they all shared: they were all fatalists, not caring about their lives and therefore unable to plan or follow through with plans, to simply achieve a better standard of living. As fatalists, we think that because we do not care about our lives, this does not mean that we do not care about the lives of others. We think that we own the right to not care for ourselves.

The fatalist in us deprives us of the imagination that could help us. Fatalists cannot imagine their spouses suffering, because the fatalists do not care. They do not see others as weak and sad. Their children feel abandoned and are therefore less confident. There is less focus in the family on education, on their children coming home with lower grades than before. Fatalists do not even notice when old friends avoid them. When they are at this stage, all decisions are fatalistic, only heightening their trauma. What follows is my own story, about how I became entrapped by this powerful feeling and how I was helped to recover.

I remember how when I was seven, I went with my mother to a nearby farmers market. On the way, my mother was holding my hand. I felt so happy, safe and proud to be her son—she was my whole world. At the market when we were buying eggs, a farmer asked me how old I was, to which I answered with pride that I was seven and in a month I was going to attend first grade. She smiled and said, "It's wonderful that you look forward to going to school. Do you know what you want to be when you grow up?"

I was happy when adults talked to me, so I answered right away: "I will be a pilot." My mother looked at me with so much love that I felt as if I could really fly. When we were back at home, she said, "I am so happy you want to be a pilot but I want you to remember that you can be whatever you decide to be."

For the next eight years, my mother kept telling me that I could be whatever I want to be. The environment where I lived, however, was telling me something quite different. I lived in a community of railroad factory workers. My father was a metal worker. When I was 14 years old, he told me to enroll in a locksmith trade school, as he had. He said, "You will not only learn there but you will also be paid because you will be working three days out of five, so you will learn how to make things."

"But Dad," I said, "I want to be a pilot."

"A pilot," he laughed. "Who put such stupid ideas into your head? Pilot training school is for those who are chosen for that, not for us. We are manual laborers, workers. You will go to trade school, the same way that others from our community do, and earn money." I said nothing but when I talked to my mother, she told me to go where my heart was telling me to go. So when I finished elementary school, I applied against my father's wishes to the most prestigious high school in our town, on track to becoming a pilot. After passing the exams, I was regarded as one of the brightest kids in the city.

My father maintained his silence at all times. On September 1, I attended class at this high school for the first time. My mother was happy, although she did not express her happiness when my father was present. The first week passed very quickly. When the second week started, it revealed what was for me an unbearable truth. Almost all the other students were more advanced than I was. Their parents, most of whom had college degrees, had helped them prepare for school even before it began, while I was still partying. The gap was obvious. In the next two weeks, I was getting Cs and Fs, while almost everyone else was getting As and Bs.

I was increasingly aware of being on the receiving end of jokes. Eventually, when I could no longer bear the situation, I stopped going to the prestigious high school and signed up for trade school, to become a locksmith. Here the situation was the opposite: I was an A student, while others were getting Fs. But that didn't make me feel better. I knew that there were others, elsewhere, much better than I, which made me increasingly depressed.

When we got paid at the end of a month, I would go with others for a drink, usually beer or wine. As the months went by, I was drinking more and more—until six months later, I was expelled from school. Thus began my life as an alcoholic. Every day, I would leave the house and meet with others like me. Together, we foraged for money to buy beer, wine or vodka. At the end of the day, I would come home drunk. I would wake up the next morning without remembering half of the previous day.

Sometimes I lost two or three days in a row, leaving home on a Friday and coming back on a Monday, thinking it was a Saturday. Thoughts of despair became more frequent and pronounced but I did not have the strength to stop them. I felt as if I was having an out-of-body experience, watching things from a distance.

One day three years later, I went to a party where I met some of my old weightlifting friends. One of them shared his story about his father throwing all of his weightlifting equipment out of the house. "I need to train but I have nowhere to go," Mirek said.

To which I responded, "You can come to my place."

"Really?" Mirek replied happily.

"Sure," I said.

What he didn't know was that, as an alcoholic, my enthusiasm was not grounded in reality. I had a very short-term perspective and I didn't remember my promises.

The next afternoon, I was napping while drunk, when I heard a loud knock on my window. I hobbled over to the window, where I saw Mirek, standing there with all his weightlifting equipment.

"What are you doing here?" I asked.

"You told me yesterday that I could bring my stuff over and we could train together."

"Well, if I said so, than come in and have fun, while I continue my nap." Of course, I didn't remember what I had promised him the day before.

After Mirek brought all his equipment into my room, he set up a bench. "Come on, let's do something together," he offered.

"Forget it," I barked.

But Mirek wouldn't give up easily. After several more attempts, he uttered the magic words: "OK, let's just do a few presses together and then we'll go for a beer, on me."

My ears perked up when I heard the word beer. I rolled over on the bed, now facing him. Mirek was sitting on the bench. All the weights were neatly placed against the wall. He looked happy. There was something very appealing about him. It was a feeling I remembered but could not pinpoint.

"Just a light workout for ten minutes and then we'll go."

"OK," I said, pulling myself out of bed.

"Lie on the bench and I'll give you the bar."

The bar felt very heavy to me after I grabbed it. I couldn't do a single press.

"Let me spot you," Mirek said, while he grabbed the bar and helped me press it several times. I felt the warmth in his voice when he spoke.

After we finished, we went for beer to a bar where we encountered some friends. We drank, talked and laughed together. After two beers, I could no longer walk straight.

"That's enough for today," Mirek said. "Let's meet again tomorrow and have some more beers." He and his friends walked me back home.

The next day when I was napping, Mirek came back and the day repeated itself. As the weeks passed, our trainings together became longer—15 minutes, 30 minutes, one hour, two hours.

After six months, I was a lot stronger. I hadn't really noticed that I was hanging out more with Mirek and his friend than with my alcoholic friends. After a year, I was as strong as Mirek. We now trained together twice daily and drank only occasionally. My mother was happy. She liked Mirek and all his friends.

I was now sober. I didn't really know how it happened. I started having conversations with neighbors and friends that I had not spoken with for many years. A new world was opening up to me, a completely new world. It was as if I had been born again.

In the spring of 1974, I began working as a fireman. That summer, I went through intensive preparation for re-entry into the high school that I had left in shame. After my application was accepted, I was overjoyed. Soon thereafter, I was confronted with an overwhelming reality. My friends who had started the same year I had were already in their second year in universities, studying to become doctors, lawyers, engineers and so on.

On the first day of school, Mirek sat together with me when the teacher welcomed and introduced everyone. I was both happy and ashamed but this time I was able to bury my shame deep inside of myself and keep studying. This time, I studied constantly and everywhere—like a mad man, greedy for knowledge: in school, in the fire department, at home, during walks, as we trained. I used every available second to catch up. Only two years earlier, I had been sleeping sometimes beside the curb, as the rainwater from the gutter washed over me, rousing me from my drunken stupor. "Hey, look, that's Jerzy," I sometimes overheard passersby saying. "What a shame. He had so much talent."

In May 1975, I finished the first year with an award. With pride, I walked over to meet Aniela, who was at the time my girlfriend, and showed her the prize, a book. In her happiness, I felt again the same warmth as I had felt from my mother and from Mirek. I also started to feel it more often, from teachers and new friends.

I had been fortunate. My alcoholic friend Jasiu, who was one year older than I, had died when he was 21. During the next few years, others had followed him.

HOPE

My Russian teacher shouted,
"Jura! You will never learn a second
language." I sat with my eyes cast down,
my cheeks burning.
After the class some students
talked to me, but I couldn't
understand them. Never,
never, never swelled in my head
like spoiled fish in a can.

I started meeting Jasiu more often.
He always kept
a bottle of wine for me.
We drank until Never

waved like worms down my body
and squeezed itself
into the cobblestones.

The last time I saw Jasiu,
he was asleep,
hugging a 12-gallon jug,
a tube in his mouth,
wine still dripping
to the cement cellar floor.

The next day, I found his last
bottle of wine and the note,
"Always yours, Jasiu."
When we buried him,
we noticed how light his coffin was,
but still we almost dropped it,
shaking on our soft legs.

How did it happen that I was spared? I had been
blessed, by people who supported me, by being there for
me—by their special kind of energy. They helped me to
move through the day with less darkness each time, until
a beam of light finally ignited in me, the light I still carry
today, a light of constant desire to improve myself and
others, circumstances notwithstanding.

I am sure you also remember a feeling inside you,
telling you that everything was good in your life. You
wake up and you are excited about the day. In the past,

you made creative decisions and you took appropriate actions to achieve your goals. Nothing that needs to be done overwhelms you, regardless of whether it requires weeks or months or even a lifetime to achieve the goals that you are ready to pursue. All strategies appear in your mind as if they were heaven sent. Planning meals and following the plan is not only easy—it is exhilarating. You cannot wait to wake up at 6 am and exercise or meditate or do whatever is necessary to improve your or someone else's life. The future is exciting and it promises even more growth. You feel good and you are happy.

Of course, there are not many moments like that in life and there are not many people who can be at this stage for a prolonged period of time but I have been blessed to know some of them.

In October 1981, I was studying engineering at the Fire Protection Academy in Warsaw. It was my last year and I was getting ready to start a new chapter in life together with my wife. The following July, I was to be sent somewhere in Poland to serve as an officer fireman. This meant that I might be living in a city I had never been to before. It also meant that I would get an apartment—a dream for young people like my wife and me. To have an apartment in Poland was almost impossible but in only eight months, we were to be in our own new apartment. I would have a good salary and it would be a perfect time to start our family. I received a list of options from which I was able to request my preferences. I preferred to be in Warsaw, where I would be able to pursue studies in chemistry, eventually earning a Ph.D.

Before coming to the Academy, I had served for five years in the fire department. My five-year delay had provided me with a wealth of experience. Usually the boys that came to the Academy came directly from high school. I, on the other hand, came with five years of experience in the fire department and the rank of senior corporal. Because of my age and my experience, I was voted leader of my class. The second year, I was elected student leader of the entire school. With my master's thesis almost completed, I was poised to begin to enjoy the fruits of my labors.

Enveloped in my dreams, I floated through the Academy as if on a flying carpet. But as my mother used to say, "Don't be so happy today—because then you will be unhappy tomorrow." It was time for events in my life to take a sharp turn. It was 1981 in Poland, at the time of the Solidarity movement. Everyone was at the same time both excited and scared. People became kind to each other, generating a feeling that the whole country was turning into one beautiful and omnipotent entity. The feeling of togetherness and courage was being awakened throughout the country.

Poland was becoming a war zone without war. Demonstrations were occurring everywhere. Thousands of people no longer scared poured out of their homes to tell the communist government, "Enough!" Hundreds of people were being arrested daily. That is when I received important news from two members of the Solidarity movement who were teachers at the Academy: Alina

Dobrowolska, who taught computer science, and Marek Surala, who taught physics. At a secret meeting, they informed me that General Wojciech Jaruzelski, whom the Russians had made president of Poland, had a plan to utilize the Academy for the purpose of defeating Solidarity. The idea was to change the status of the Academy from a public to a paramilitary organization. This would have enabled Jaruzelski to utilize the fire department to quell demonstrations.

I had a very uneasy feeling inside, a feeling that I was about to lose everything I had worked toward, both professionally and personally. But the alternative, of not doing anything to oppose this plan, was even worse. "What can we do?" I asked.

"I don't know," Marek said.

"I don't know if you are willing to risk your position but in my opinion, you should tell all the students the truth," Alina said.

"You know what will happen if I do that. I will be blacklisted."

"It's your call," Marek added. "Whatever you do is up to you. We fulfilled our responsibility and now it is time for you to fulfill yours."

"Okay," I said. "I will talk to the heads of each year's class and will see what they want to do."

After a short discussion, all student leaders decided to inform all the students about the situation. At the meeting, some four hundred student firemen decided to initiate a peaceful protest. Even though the protest was innocent, it disturbed many officers whose responsibility was to keep the students uninformed and pacified. But the officers were losing their grip over the students from the first and second years who lived on the Academy campus.

When the officers fired shots at 10 pm on November 25 in 1981, I ordered an emergency meeting of all students. The third and fourth year students lived one hour from the Academy. When we arrived, the gate was locked. We were unable to enter the building without assistance. We asked Solidarity members to help us. After about an hour, Marek Holuszko, together with some workers from the Warsaw Steel factory, came to help by supporting and by witnessing the present situation, to prevent violence from breaking out.

Seeing the overwhelming support received from Solidarity members, the officers on duty opened the gate of the Academy, allowing us to gather in the main lecture hall. After an hour, all students voted in favor of an occupied strike and I announced that the strike had begun.

The next day, no one could enter the building. All teachers and staff stood outside. The police arrived, as did more Solidarity members. Police set up a fence around the building, preventing anyone from entering. Thousands of people, including students' parents, came to support us, with food and moral support. At the end of the day, it was clear to everyone that we would not back down unless the school was allowed to maintain its status as a strictly civilian organization.

Negotiations began with the government. To help us deal with an increasingly intense situation, three particular individuals came to help. Seweryn Jaworski, who represented Solidarity, ensured direct communication with Solidarity headquarters in Warsaw. Kazimierz Wejchert, a professor at Warsaw Polytechnic University, helped us formulate our demands in correct legal language. Jerzy Popieluszko, a priest, came from the Church of St. Kostki to offer us moral and spiritual support.

When Wejchert and Jaworski came, it was obvious to me that they had one purpose: the establishment of a free and independent Poland. I was extremely impressed with these two men and did everything I could to be around them and learn as much as I could from them.

At first, I could not imagine that anyone could be more inspiring than these two men but I was wrong. Jerzy Popieluszko was even more amazing. He had a calm and loving presence, emanating peacefulness, free of aggressiveness or anxiety. In his presence, my fears and worries about the future dissipated. I was 27 at that time and it was the first time I encountered someone who loved me unconditionally. No matter how my disbelief tried to discredit the possibility of being loved simply because I was a human being, it could not succeed. For the next ten days and nights, I lived on coffee and cigarettes, without sleeping. Unfortunately, after ten days of negotiations, the Polish government decided to end our strike by force. Police stormed the building from the ground, while a special antiterrorist brigade used helicopters to land on the roof. They found four hundred of us gathered in the main hall, after which they announced that the academy no longer existed. We were ordered to leave the building. We were also presented with an option to swear allegiance to the new school, if we wanted to continue our studies.

THE LAST FIRE

"Government gives Fire Academy to the army,"
the broadcast said while I was cleaning a ladder;
I sat down and held my head between my hands
covered with ashes from last night's fire.

I was one semester
from graduating to fulfill
my childhood dream—I was five
the first time I ran out of the house
after hearing a fire siren.
Without waving my hands,
I stood still at the curb looking
at the passing truck—I wanted to be
inside a fireman's uniform,
to become a friend of fires,
to crawl between flames.

But the broadcast meant
I would have to color water
to spray Solidarity demonstrators
so they could be recognized and arrested.

We marched by the hundreds
to the lecture hall
and raised our fists,
"NO!"

The next day, policemen surrounded the school
while our families, steel factory workers,
and professors stood behind them in the snow,
trying to pass
a cigarette, an apple.

Each evening we prayed with Popieluszko,
the patron of the Warsaw Steel Factory,
who filled us with enough courage
to close our eyes at night.

On the tenth morning,
pieces from broken doors burst
ahead of policemen who kicked us
till they'd warmed their cold feet.

We were given one chance to swear
allegiance to the new school
governed by Jaruzelski's comrades.
We didn't even consider it—
they loaded us into buses
and drove away between soldiers
gathered around tanks.

But we weren't scared,
we just looked behind them
to where our empty fire engines
stood in the garage.

Sometimes, today, even in my forties
I want to jump onto
a passing fire truck, tie my
uniform whose sleeves still smell
of the last fire around my sweaty skin,
but instead I stand with my eyes
on the line of the horizon
where I saw the last blue light
flashing—the sound of a siren still
caressing my dry ears.

Even though I loved being a fireman, I decided
together with more than a hundred others not to swear
allegiance to a new Fire Protection Academy, focusing on
helping other students to get into different schools and
find them support while they studied. My underground
experience began in Jerzy Popieluszko's church. To be
close to Jerzy was a blessing. Whenever I met him, I felt
as if I got a shot of love. Millions of other Poles felt the
same way. Jerzy's sermons became increasingly powerful
because of their power of love. Unfortunately, the leaders
of the Polish government could not stand it anymore.
On October 19, 1984, four policemen kidnaped Jerzy,
tortured him and threw his body into a river.

EVEN IN THE ICY RIVER

Every morning I walked into the church
where Jerzy Popieluszko,
the Warsaw Steel Factory priest,
prayed with the workers.
Usually, at the beginning of a sermon,
he lifted his eyelids and kept looking
until the silence brought us back from yesterday.
Then he covered his hollowed cheeks
with his long fingers and began,
"Love. Open our fists."

He traveled from one church to another
but one day in the early morning
four policemen stopped his car.
They threw his body into the trunk
and drove to the nearby forest
where they hit him
with metal clubs, screaming,
"Open our fists,
open our fists!
Where is your love?"

They couldn't see that he had already left,
that he kept his head down praying for them
even when they tightened a rope
around his feet and attached rocks,
even when they cut his stomach,
and even when they threw his body into the icy river.
The river we drink water from.

The loss to the Polish people was overwhelming. I fell into a deep depression and could not come out of it. Spending weeks in the church did not help. In February 1985, I was still depressed, so when I was ordered to come for an interrogation to the police station in Szczecin, I did not care if anything happened to me. The next day at the police station, I was sent to a big room to wait my turn. There were maybe fifty other people waiting, as I sat on a bench and began reading a book. After several minutes, a man came into the room. I recognized my close friend Mietek, from the Szczecin Olympic Weightlifting team. Together with Otto and Wojtek, Mietek and I were close friends, always training together and having fun. I rushed over to him and shook his hand. We were happy for a moment, the intervening years seemingly irrelevant. He was the first to break our joy. "What are you doing here?" he asked.

I told him my story about studying fire protection engineering.

Then I asked him, "What have you been doing?" He looked at me with a strange kind of gaze I had never seen before, one that made me feel uncomfortable.

"No," I said.

"Yes," he said, "I became an officer some years ago." Then he added, "Let me find out what is going on with you." He took my paper and went through a nearby door. After a few minutes, he returned with my paper. "It's not good. I was able to cover up for you. Don't come back here ever again. If you do, you will never leave."

"Are you sure about that?" I asked.

"Yes," he said. "I am sure. You had been assigned to me."

"So that means ... ?" I stopped myself, before completing the sentence. Mietek was silent.

I shook his hand and said, "What a life this is, eh?"

When I told my wife the story, she said, "It's clear that you have to leave the country now. I will stay behind, so they don't suspect that you are escaping."

I left Poland as soon as I was able to obtain a passport, a few weeks later, on March 8, International Women's Day, probably the happiest day in Poland. On this day, all women are showered with flowers and gifts. Everyone is friendly with each other, even when they are not acquainted, and everyone nurtures one another.

I said goodbye to Aniela that day, without knowing when we would see each other again. In Sweden, I immediately checked into the Solidarity headquarters in Stockholm, where I learned that my depression was minor in comparison with others. People like me were separated from their loved ones. Husbands waited for years for their wives and children to join them but the Polish government would not release them, suspecting the whole family would stay abroad permanently. Keeping families apart was a form of punishment.

Usually situations like these ended in hunger strikes. Sometimes a man whose family was still in Poland would sit in front of the Polish Embassy for days without food and would eventually be reunited with his family. Sometimes he would be taken to a hospital because of weakness and exhaustion.

The suffering of Polish people in Stockholm moved

and inspired me to help. Instead of complaining about my own situation, I began helping others by supporting them with inspiring words. As I talked with people, I began to experience a feeling similar to when I was traveling in a fire truck to a fire scene for the first time. I felt proud that someone somewhere needed me and I was going to help. More and more people came to my place and asked me to help them sort things out.

People started calling me a village priest, which could not have made me happier. One day, a psychologist from Poland named Wanda Saj came to me for help. After several meetings, she said, "You have a certain clarity when you talk. I don't know how to describe it but it is very helpful. I encourage you strongly to write."

"Write?" I asked. "Why should I write?"

"Because you have something to offer and you should care enough to pass it along to others."

I was speechless. My mind was racing. In Poland, I was always a scientist and never an artist. All books that I had ever read were about science.

Wanda patiently awaited my answer.

"But I have never written anything," I said. "How could I write without having learned how?"

"It's not important how you write. What's important is that you do it," she said, with a pleasant smile.

"Okay," I said, "I will try."

"Don't try," she said. "Just do it. Write."

It was almost midnight when I came back to my hotel room. I sat at my desk, took out a pen and stared at a blank page. No thoughts came to me. Nothing important was happening in my head. I closed my eyes and spent about twenty minutes sitting silently. My whole life was rolling in front of me as if I was in a movie theater.

When it ended, I opened my eyes and wrote the first word: "Rebirth." Then I started writing sentences. After writing two sentences, it became clear that I was writing a poem, even though I had never read one in my entire life. I thought for a moment that this may be temporary but as I turned the page and kept writing, it continued to be verse.

When I met Wanda the next day, I gave her the poem. She looked at it, then at me and back at the poem, after which she said, "I knew that there was something about you that I couldn't grasp, but now I see it. You are a poet."

I laughed and said, "Just writing a poem does not make me a poet. To be a poet, one needs to have a life calling for this."

"You will have such a calling. I'm sure about that."

"Well, I don't know about that. There are more important things on my mind right now than writing poetry."

"You will do important things and you will also write poetry. About this, I am certain. I feel it. And I think that you should stay in Sweden and we should open a practice together, so you can continue helping people."

I liked Wanda and I didn't know how to tell her that I was not going to stay but it seemed she already knew.

"You intend to leave, right?"

"Yes, I have to," I said.

"Why? Sweden is a beautiful country. There are many people that need your gift and you will have plenty of time to write poetry."

"You see," I said, "when I was 15, someone asked me where I was born, meaning where in Poland. But when I wanted to answer, I had a feeling that I didn't really belong there." At that point, I wondered whether I should continue.

"You can tell me," Wanda said, reassuringly. "Everything is safe with me." Wanda had a very inviting and harmless nature. I trusted her.

"Well, my body was born in Poland but my mind ...." I hesitated for a moment. Without knowing why, I said, "But I feel as if my mind was not born in Poland."

Wanda was looking deep inside me and said, "In America, right?"

I was surprised. "How did you know?"

"I have seen it before. I hoped that maybe you could find a home here but you have to liberate yourself and become independent before you will find peace and devote yourself to a higher purpose."

I didn't understand what she meant by a higher purpose but I was glad she agreed with my calling.

I was able to leave Sweden faster than I thought I would be able to. Within a week, I received a phone call from the CIA office in Munich, Germany. The Warsaw underground, especially people that were involved in the strike and Radio Solidarity, experienced many arrests. I was called to Munich to help identify the spy within the underground, the person responsible for the arrests.

During the next three weeks at the CIA office in Munich, I revealed what I knew, hoping that this would contribute to identifying the spy within the movement. Shortly afterward, my wife and I were granted status as political refugees in the US. With $1,000 in savings and one huge piece of luggage, we landed at JFK Airport in New York. We then boarded another plane for Detroit, where our sponsoring company was located.

Although we made it to our destination, our luggage unfortunately did not. It was somehow lost, never to be found. Aniela looked very upset, so I told her that maybe God wants us to discard everything from the old country and begin a completely new life here. This at least seemed to offer her a certain degree of comfort, seeing how calm I was.

During our stay in Germany, we had befriended Andrzej, who was now in Los Angeles and offered help if we wanted to relocate there. In the morning, we said goodbye to our sponsors in Detroit and took a taxi to the airport. The tickets to LA cost us $400, leaving us with only $600 and the clothes on our backs. As our plane approached Los Angeles at 11 pm, the city was illuminated below us. It was magical to see so many lights. Even pools were lit. I was mesmerized by the beauty and the power.

Aniela looked worried, so I said, "In two years, we will have a house with a pool, too." That was a mistake. Aniela looked at me as if I had lost my mind. Years later, she admitted that she really thought so. For the next two weeks, we were preoccupied with survival. We slept on the floor in different homes almost every day. Later, a kind Polish family who lived in Los Feliz let us sleep in the unfinished second house they were building. It was cold but it was where we found our first home in America. We warmed each other under three blankets and dreamed about having our own place.

After two weeks, I was rejected for employment by a fire department. I was told that, at 32, I was too old and overqualified, in terms of both education and experience. A month passed and I still could not find a job. With the idea of utilizing my expertise as an Olympic weightlifting coach, I made an appointment with Bob Hise, president of the AWA (American Weightlifting Association) and went to see him in Eagle Rock. Bob was a great man. People loved him and obviously respected him. I told him who I was and asked about any opportunity to make a living doing training for Olympic Weightlifting. "There is no money in weightlifting," he said. "All coaches who come from Eastern Block countries open auto repair or body shops and make a very good living at it. If you want to fix cars I can introduce you to some of them."

"I don't want to fix cars," I said.

Bob thought for a moment and said, "There's a new trend in gyms with something called personal trainers, which is something you could try. But Olympic weight-lifting coaches don't like to work with regular people, so I don't know if you would like that but you could try."

"Where could I find such a gym?" I asked.

"I don't know," Bob said, "but you could look around and eventually find one. You don't need a car."

My wife and I walked in increasingly larger circles from where we were staying in Los Feliz. One day, we arrived at a place called Power Source in Burbank. After I introduced myself to Aram, the owner, I asked about the possibility of working in the gym as a personal trainer.

"The best I could do for you is to hire you for a one-week trial period. I would pay you $5 an hour and you would work five hours a day, for five days." Aram shook my hand and wished me luck.

"But what exactly should I do?" I asked. Aram smiled and said, "I really don't know. You'll have to figure that out as you go. You have a week to make it work."

Aniela was happy. "You got a job!" she said, hugging me. "But you will need gym shoes," she added. We found the nearest Salvation Army outlet and walked inside. The only gym shoes that fit me cost a dollar but they happened to be pink. I bought them. The next day, in my bright pink shoes, I stood in the gym, ready for my new career. Jimmy, a manger, knew about me and greeted me with a big smile that got even broader after he saw my shoes.

"What should I do?" I asked.

"Well," Jimmy said, "If someone new comes to the gym, he will get a free session with you and your job will be to help him become familiar with the gym equipment. If he has any questions about health or fitness, you will do your best to help him.

"If he likes what you've done for him, he may want some private sessions with you. If a person buys a session, he will pay us $25, of which 60 percent will be yours."

I immediately calculated that I could earn $15 an hour, which was a lot of money for me at the time. The first person who was referred to me reported back pains and said he wanted to lose weight. I created a daily routine for him, to make his back more flexible and I designed a food plan so he could lose weight.

The next person referred to me had high cholesterol and high blood pressure. I also created for her a specific exercise routine and a food plan. The next referral was a model who wanted a more attractive and agile body. I also designed a plan for her to follow so she could achieve her goals.

After a few hours, there were no new referrals, so I looked around the gym for anyone who looked if he or she needed help. In the far corner of the gym, I spotted two men in their early 30s doing deadlifts. They were both about 6-foot-4 and 300 pounds. Both of them were lifting 315 pounds. It was obvious to me that although they were big, they were weak for their size and had very poor lifting technique, which would prevent them from getting stronger. They rounded their backs, to compensate for their weak leg muscles. If they continued this way, they would end up with stronger backs but even weaker legs, which would eventually lead to herniated discs.

I walked directly over to them to tell them. They stared down at my five-foot, six-inch frame, weighing only 130 pounds and wearing pink shoes. I felt that if I didn't do something dramatic, they would grab me by my shirt and carry me out of the gym. So I walked over to the bar that was loaded with 315 pounds and said, "Here: Let me show you."

Surprised and amused, they decided to watch and see what would happen. The weight was heavy even for them and of course they couldn't imagine that I could lift it off the ground. I grabbed the bar and lifted it six times, in rapid succession, about one second for each rep. After I set the bar down, I said, "If you lift like this instead, your legs will get stronger and you'll avoid injuring your back."

They just stood there, dumbfounded, without saying anything. In the absence of any response, I walked over to the reception area, to see whether there were any new referrals for me.

The next day, the two men approached me to thank me and to shake my hand. I later learned that they were both night club bouncers. Years later, this connection came in handy, as they introduced us to other bouncers, who spared us from waiting in long lines.

The news about my ability to enable people to become stronger, lose weight or get off medications spread quickly throughout the gym and beyond. New people coming to the gym were asking specifically for me. I was soon working fourteen hours a day, seven days a week. Almost overnight, I lost my fear of not having enough money. My wife had a very similar experience.

We worked, worked and worked. Two years passed by very quickly. One day, a client of ours named Karl Angel asked me whether I go out. "Go out?" I asked. "What do you mean by that?"

"I mean go out for dinner?"

"No," I said. "We have never been out for dinner here. We eat at home."

"Well," he said, "let me introduce you to a great place. It's Italian and the restaurant has been operated by the same family for three generations."

"No," I said. "We do not want to go."

Karl looked at me and said, "Come on, let me take you there. It will be fun."

For some reason, I didn't want to disappoint him, so I agreed.

Saturday evening, dressed as if going to a wedding, we were picked up by Karl and his wife, Lisset.

The restaurant was great. All the food looked fantastic and was delicious. It was the first time that I had gnocchi. I always liked anything cooked with potatoes and my mother cooked a very similar dish, called kopytka. This was our first time in an American restaurant and when time came to pay, Karl—who knew how hard we worked and how difficult it was for us to live—tried to prepare me for his paying for our dinner. Of course he knew how that could be difficult because I took pride in being independent. So when he offered to pay for us I said absolutely not. He made a couple more attempts but finally gave up after it was apparent that I would not accept.

This experience had a big effect on us. We realized that people here have a different approach to life and it would be good for us to go out sometimes. So whenever we had time, we would go out for breakfast together and we enjoyed being served.

Food was sometimes a topic of conversation when I trained my clients, so when Thomas Griffith found out that we had never eaten sushi, he insisted on inviting us to his favorite sushi bar. This time it was easier for me to agree. The next day, he and his wife, Mary, picked us up and took us to the restaurant. Of course, they ordered everything and the first thing I tasted was white tuna albacore. Thomas and Mary watched when I put the piece of sushi into my mouth. It was soft, warm and very tasty. My expression when swallowing prompted them to shout, "Yes, yes!" My wife loved sushi, too, and we ate a lot that day. When the time came to pay, Thomas said, "Let me treat you guys. It would be my pleasure." This time it was easy for me to simply say thank you. Slowly, we were becoming Americans, working hard and enjoying our lives.

In 1989, everybody talked about houses, the values of which were increasing virtually overnight. It seemed that if we didn't buy right away, we would never be able to afford a home. We didn't have enough money for a down payment but some of our clients offered to pay us in advance for six months of services.

Karl helped us find a real estate agent and we were ready to find our first home. When I talked to my client Pat Wallace about our intention, she suggested that we rent rather than buy. "Houses are now overpriced," she said. "They will decline in value within a year or two. Why not wait a while? Save up some more money and you will have your house soon."

But the prospect of having our own home in combination with other people's anxiety about this was keeping us up at night. Our emotions and imagination were driving us to buy, in spite of some warning signs that the time was not right.

Our agent found us a home in Van Nuys, a three-bedroom fixer-upper with a pool. My dream was coming true. The house was listed for $220,000 and when we asked our agent how we should proceed, she said that we should offer full price if we like the home and want to buy it, even though it needed a lot of work. In six weeks, escrow closed and we had the keys in our hands, as we walked with our client Chris Huntley for the first time into our new home.

When I opened the door, I was reminded that it smelled terribly and it was dirty. Everything from the roof to the floor had to be replaced. When we were outside after seeing everything, I said, "Well, in a month, we will have a big party." Both Aniela and Chris looked at me as if I had lost my mind. Indeed, it took us a whole year and about $40,000 to fix it but it certainly looked beautiful—white with black trim and a red door—dressed in bougainvillea, above the front entrance.

Our housewarming party was a blast. Probably two hundred people showed up and brought all kind of things we needed for our house, as well as all the food for the potluck. We enjoyed the house immensely, inviting many of our clients, who became our friends. Life became stable and we saw the promise of a great future ahead of us.

Even though we could not imagine that anything bad would happen to us, the depression of 1990 came, bringing with it the collapse of real estate values. Almost overnight, our home's value dropped 50 percent, to $110,000. For the next few years, we concentrated on working and paying the bills. After five years, however, the negative situation began to take its toll on us.

We visited our bank to propose to sell the house based on the current market value. But the bank representative told us that this is not the way business is done in America and if we wanted to keep the house, we needed to continue to make our payments. I suggested that if the house was foreclosed on, the bank would probably lose even more money but that didn't change anything. The banker simply answered that if they allowed us to do that, everyone else would want to lower their payments and the lender would lose too much money.

Drained by the whole situation, we decided to let the house go into foreclosure, even though some of our clients suggested that we rent it out and wait for values to come back. We thought about it but we didn't have the energy for that and chose instead to return to apartment living, as tenants. So it was that we moved from Van Nuys to an apartment in Marina Del Rey.

We needed new purpose and motivation, to find meaning in life after losing everything that we had worked for during the past ten years. Back to where we had started a decade ago, we tried to comprehend what had just happened. The only solution seemed to be to move forward.

Our desire for emotional and spiritual recovery prompted us to enter the MFA program in creative writing at Vermont College, with an emphasis in poetry. We also started competing in Masters Weightlifting championships and we formed an Olympic Weightlifting Team at Gold's Gym in Venice, California. School, competition, work and coaching took our minds off of thinking about the past, about thinking of losing our home and our sense of security.

We graduated in 1998 with MFA degrees in creative writing. Two years earlier, we had competed in the 1996 World Weightlifting championship in Canada, with Aniela winning gold and me silver. We competed in Poland at the weightlifting championship in 1997, winning two gold medals. In 1998, because I was injured, I did not enter the Nike World Masters Games. Aniela did and won the games. In 1999, we went to Scotland, where we both won the Masters World Weightlifting championship. That year, we moved our team to UCLA and founded the UCLA weightlifting team, registering it with United States Weightlifting Federation in Colorado Springs. Some members of the team entered the State Weightlifting Championship in 2004. Walter Chi won state championship and Michael Casey came in third.

Two thousand four was another year of great change for us. After 25 years, we were blessed with a pregnancy, with Aniela expecting in August. Michelle and David Kelly, who were moving to Woodside, told us that it would be a wonderful place to raise our child. We drove there the next weekend, to have a look. As soon as we drove into the village, we were in love with Woodside.

We could not afford to live there, however, unless we could borrow money toward a down payment for a new home. With Aniela five months pregnant, we relived the scenario from 15 years before, putting together a down payment with the help of our clients, who advanced us six months of fees for services. We made the purchase in June and moved in on the Fourth of July, at 2 am.

Natalie was born on August 16 and I was working very hard again to pay our bills. Most of our clients were in Los Angeles, so for the next two years, we drove to Los Angeles every Friday, after seeing clients in Woodside, to spend the weekend in Southern California. Aniela, Natalie and I were staying at a Studio City guesthouse that two of our clients, Madeleine and Jeffrey Tucker, were kind enough to let us use. We would see some of our clients at the guesthouse, while we would drive to the homes of others.

On Monday, I would coach the UCLA weightlifting team until 11:30 am, after which we would drive back to Woodside, where I would see my first client there at 5:30 pm. Week after week for the next two years, this was our life. Our fear of failure gradually diminished, as our client roster in Woodside steadily grew. During drive time, we wrote *The Happy Body* book, which was published in 2009. The next five years were concentrated on helping people achieve *The Happy Body* lifestyle.

I noticed that even though people knew what was good for them and had plans and a strategy to achieve it, they would easily jeopardize their efforts by following destructive habits. It became clear to me that people need inspiration. Whenever someone allowed the voice of the Fatalist to dominate, it would destroy what the individual wanted to create. I wrote a poem to help them to identify not with the voice of the Fatalist but with that of the Master, who is able to do what we often do not like but is nonetheless good for us. After five years, I had written 56 poems, which I later published under the title, *A Healthy Mirror for Change: Nourishing an Appetite for Losing Weight*. These poems proved very helpful in fighting destructive decisions.

During the past year, I realized that my clients were expressing themselves in strongly contradictory voices. Just five minutes after committing to losing weight,

someone would say that it would be impossible. I began identifying internal dialogues that go on within us.
In so doing, I helped my clients to see that we are not destined to a certain way of living, that how we live is the result of our decisions. I learned that there is a constant dialogue within us and that dialogue is between two opposing forces: the Fatalist and the Master. The one that dominates shapes our life.

As I explored the language of these two dominant forces within us, I increasingly came to the realization that there is a natural tendency to identify with the Master (a heroic, positive force) and turn away from the Fatalist. Even if initially only for a moment, this energy accumulates over time to the point that it eventually begins to effect a transformation, by means of internal dialogue.

As I watched people change in their orientation from Fatalist to Master, I noticed changes in the way they use language. In the first week of practicing *The Happy Body*, practitioners report choosing the wrong foods or food amounts, without any real awareness of doing it, as if their knowledge of what was right was suspended during the time that the transgressions are committed. People on the program who are unable to lose weight become disappointed, frustrated and unhappy.

When they are in the second week of the program, they report being aware of choosing the wrong foods but they feel as if they are watching the scenario from the outside, rather than exercising control over what happens. During this phase, certain individuals are still unable to lose weight, even though they experience a weak positive voice that gives them hope.

In the third week, they report having an internal debate that could sometimes go on for minutes, before either the Fatalist or Master within them prevails. One day, it might be the Fatalist within them that prevails. Another day, it may be the Master. The situation is fluid, capable of changing within minutes. People in this phase could follow the program perfectly for three days—and then fail for two—or any combination (3-4, 5-2, 7-3 or whatever). They usually lose three pounds and gain the weight back or they sometimes go on like this, back and forth, for months. They lose 30 or 40 pounds over time and then gain them back, obliged to begin anew.

The fourth week is usually a breakthrough. People still have an internal conversation but this time the Master within them is much stronger in terms of contributing to the decision. At this point, practitioners know that they are improving and happy to share this with others. They are still afraid of gaining weight, although the voice of the Fatalist at this time is weak, without the power to prompt the individual to regain weight. Upon entering my studio, these people are beaming with pride and happiness. They know they are changing for the better and that nothing threatens this progress.

In the fifth week, practitioners stop experiencing the negative voice of the Fatalist altogether. All decisions are positive and constructive. As they no longer need my services with regard to weight loss, I ask them to become more independent, coming only occasionally or whenever they really need supplemental information relating to the program.

As I analyzed my clients' situations in terms of failures relating to losing weight, thereby becoming disappointed and unhappy, I identified 12 common challenging situations. I then wrote five-level dialogues between Fatalist and Master, in response to these situations.

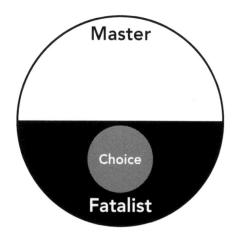

The first level, which I call Fatalist, is dominated completely by the voice of the Fatalist. A person in this situation needs outside help because there is no help offered by the Master, who is entirely absent from the internal dialogue. When I was an alcoholic, I could not pull myself out of the addiction without outside help from Mirek. On a daily basis, Mirek channeled the voice of the Master for me.

In my thirties, when I ate food from a plate or bowl or pot, I would keep eating until I finished everything, even if my stomach hurt. On one occasion, Aniela videotaped me. A fruit salad was left after a party we gave. The contents of the large wooden bowl easily exceeded ten pounds. I sat outside, with the bowl between my legs, as I began eating. When I watched the video, I noticed that I didn't take my gaze off the contents of the bowl, even for a second. It was only after I had finished that I lifted my head, at which time I saw Aniela filming. She laughed as if she had been watching an entertaining comedy. This was the first time that I consciously became aware of my eating habit.

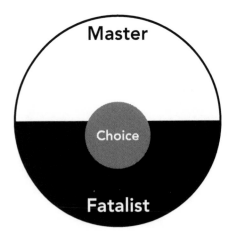

The second level, which I refer to as the Disbeliever, represents the relative strength of Fatalist as 75% and the Master as 25%. A person at this level cannot make a positive choice even though it is provided. When I was buying a home, Pat was the voice of the Master, showing me the best choice for me at the time. I was blinded, however, by the voice within me of the Fatalist, who was impatient and could not wait. When we lived in Marina Del Rey, we had a weekly all-you-can-eat Sunday buffet brunch at The Warehouse Restaurant on Admiralty Way. We usually arrived before 10 am, the first diners to enter. There were tables outside with a clear view of water and sailboats. It was beautiful. We sat there and usually enjoyed the scenery for a while, as we drank champagne. Then we began our trips to the inside where we found the food: steak, potatoes, fish, pork chops, mushrooms and so on. Stomach pains usually began after an hour, with the Master within us suggesting that we either pause or stop eating altogether, as we had already gotten our money's worth. But the voice of the Fatalist was too strong. We just kept on eating, finishing three hours later, at 1 pm, with coffee and the last piece of my favorite, tiramisu cake. We lived close by, so in five minutes, we were back in our apartment. After another five minutes, we fell into a sleeping stupor, snoring for another several hours. We would usually wake up at 5 pm, groggy and surprised by where the day had gone.

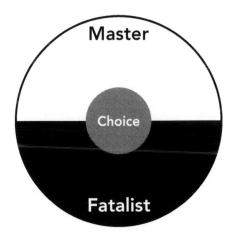

The third level, which I call the Debater, happens when the Fatalist and the Master carry equal influence. At this level, it is difficult to make a decision. Usually we struggle until we are tired and our willpower is weak, at which the outcome can go either way.

In 2002, we lived in Santa Monica, where we loved to go for dinner to a friend's restaurant, La Vecchia Cucina. There they baked a delicious, crispy homemade Panini bread. The bread would come out steaming hot from the oven, after which it was offered with olive oil, basil and garlic, which we would scoop up in large quantities using the bread. Usually before we ate anything else, we had two or three loaves of Panini bread, by which time we were full. But we ordered food anyway, so as not to offend the waiter.

One day, Aniela suggested we go there but I refused. "The bread is too powerful. If I go there, I will come back seven pounds heavier."

Aniela shrugged her shoulders. "Okay," she said. "We can always stay home and make dinner ourselves." She went to the kitchen and started looking for ingredients.

I went to the office and paced like a tiger, back and forth, as my internal dialogue proceeded: "I love the restaurant but I cannot go there. This is ridiculous. I must go and conquer the bread. It is either me or the bread that will emerge the winner. Today, I will conquer the bread. I cannot allow the bread to be stronger than I am. How is it possible that bread could be stronger than a poet, a teacher, a world weightlifting champion?"

So we decided to go. When I entered the restaurant, I seated myself immediately at the bar. Mark the bartender usually worked on Friday evenings and gave us our customary drinks. Without any hesitation, he poured my favorite drink, vodka with fresh lime. I called this drink a foggy. As Mark brought out the bread with olive oil and extra basil and garlic, I was just finishing my drink. I put the glass down and asked Mark to refill it. Then, with one hand, I grabbed one piece of bread and inhaled its fragrance deeply. With the other hand, I held my hand with the bread, preventing myself from putting the bread into my mouth. It was difficult but it worked.

With my second drink, I repeated the action with the bread. This time, it was much easier to resist. The third time, I just smelled it—without holding my arm, as I had seen Russian weightlifters do—and put it back. I don't know what happened with my brain but the bread had lost its power over me and the game was over. We returned to this restaurant many times, without stuffing ourselves with the bread. The Master within me had triumphed.

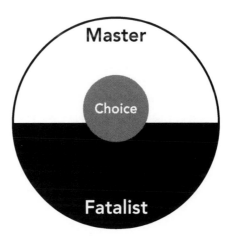

The fourth level, which I have named the Hesitator, represents the strength of the Fatalist at 25% and the Master at 75%. A person on this level makes a positive choice even though the voice of the Fatalist tries to dissuade against making the right choice. When Michelle and David told us that Woodside would be a great place for our daughter, Natalie, to grow up, we made the decision to move there even though our entire clientele was located in the Los Angeles area, where many friends also lived. In short, we loved the area and felt it would be a tremendous sacrifice to leave but the welfare of our child was more important.

In 1997, four days before leaving for Scotland to compete in the Masters World Weightlifting championship, Marek and Malgosia Probosz celebrated Marek's birthday and invited us to the party. We adored them but with only four days before the competition, any intake of excess food would put us at risk of weighing too much and therefore dehydrating our bodies just hours before competition, thereby running the risk of becoming too weak and forfeiting our chance of winning. When I told Aniela that we could attend the party, she said: "Of course we can go. We have to go and be able to have fun with these guys, as we do the right thing for ourselves. We need to learn to cope with such challenges."

I wanted to go, so I said: "Okay, let's go."

Aware of our situation, Malgosia and Marek didn't expect us. So when we showed up, they were extremely happy. The voices of our Masters within us were strong. We ate only what we needed, as we engaged in conversation and dancing. We hadn't even noticed that five hours had passed and it was time to go home.

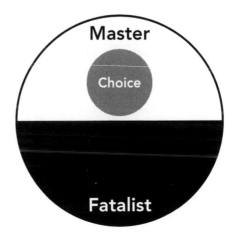

The fifth and last level, which I call the Master, is dominated 100% by the voice of the Master. At this level, we don't make any negative or destructive decisions. As my body ages and my metabolic rate drops, my body requires less food, so I simply adapt to the amount my body needs. In so doing, I avoid all the disappointment, frustration and suffering involved with gaining excess weight.

After living for sixty years, I have learned that most of our decisions are about simple things we do on a daily basis like eating a bagel or drinking a glass of juice, going to a movie or staying home. These decisions are so rooted in the past that it is impossible for us to change anything unless we change our past. We eat more then we need to because that's what we did in the past. We spend hours each day on the Internet because that's what we have done in the past. There are other decisions that can affect our lives negatively.

Had I not left Poland, would I still be alive? This is something I will never know. Some decisions, on the other hand, have definite negative repercussions. The pain of loss with which they are associated makes it difficult to forget these things. After we lost our home, whenever I dwelled on it, I became depressed. Even today, after many years have passed, I still think about what might have been if I hadn't bought the home that I lost or if I had bought it after the economic downturn, for $110,000, instead of the $220,000 I had paid for it before the crash. My life would be so less painful and I would not have found myself fifteen years later in the same position, without a home, borrowing money to buy another dream home.

We tend to make choices based on our past, with intuition developed from past experiences. But in order to make the decisions that are best for ourselves, we must break free of the past. Since we cling to our past—and all the choices we make are based on our intuition—we are unable to create a better past for ourselves. We need to be aware of our situation and choose what our past does not like but it is good for us. We must make conscious choices until they become our past and our intuition develops from this "new" past.

This book will enable you, first, to identify the voices of the Fatalist and the Master within you. Second, it will help you to become conscious about the voices, by writing your own dialogues. Third, it will empower you with ability to apply what you have learned in actual situations, observing not only the Fatalist and Master within you but also within others.

How to Use This Book

This book was written to make your life better, by making you aware of the different voices that speak within you while dealing with exercise. First, you will become aware that you have voices, so you will not have to depend anymore on believing in destiny. As soon as you become aware of these voices, you will start to recognize them in the dialogues. Second, after you are able to recognize the voices, you will start practicing to write your own dialogues. After practicing all the dialogues, you will gain the ability to realize that any situation creates a power struggle within us and that you will be able to direct this struggle to the constructive outcome by leaning toward the Master. As soon as you gain this ability to choose the Master within you, you will be able to recognize the voices outside of yourself— in your friends, family members, as well as strangers— and you will be able to help them to become aware and guide them to work with themselves to achieve this life-changing power, reflected in the voice of the Master.

First, read the dialogues and become aware of your inner dialogues. Second, practice writing all the dialogues provided in Part II: Practice Writing Dialogues. Third, after you have developed the ability to write out all these dialogues, start applying them to real life. Go for example to a dinner with friends and listen to your inner voices, as well as to those of others. As soon as you are able to consciously recognize all the different voices within you and within others, you will become liberated from both the Fatalist within you and the Fatalist in others.

For ease of reading, the voice of the (slanted, distorted) Fatalist is represented in italics, while that of the (upright, balanced) Master is non-italicized.

Part I
Identify the Voices Within

WAKING UP

Scenario 1. Jen is sleeping. It is 6 AM and the alarm just went off to remind her to go to the gym and workout.

I. Fatalist:

"I am too tired, so I will sleep for another hour and do my workout in the evening."

II. Disbeliever:

"I am too tired, so I will sleep for another hour and do my workout in the evening."

"It will make you feel better."

"Yes, I know, but I am too tired."

"You only have the feeling that you are tired, but really you are rested. You just slept for nine hours."

"I cannot do anything about it. If I'm tired, I sleep."

"Maybe you had too much sleep, so you're tired."

"There is never enough sleep."

II. Debater:

"I am too tired, so I will sleep for another
hour and do my workout in the evening."

"Stop whining and get up."

"I don't whine; I'm just tired."

"Are you kidding me? You slept for nine hours."

"I can't do anything about my lack of energy."

"If you exercised everyday, you'd have more energy."

"The reason everything that happens to me is bad
is that I don't exercise enough.
Wouldn't you agree that sometimes it can just be
a lack of sleep or missing a nutrient in my body?"

"Did you forget that you sleep nine or ten hours a day,
and you are fifty pounds overweight?"

"What does being overweight have to do with being tired?"

"How can a person who is fifty pounds overweight
miss any nutrient at all?

"For you everything seems logical,
but for me there are many inexplicable

reasons why I'm sluggish all day long."

"You just don't want to admit that
you will do anything so you don't have to exercise."

"That's not true, and I will prove it to you tomorrow."

"Tomorrow. There is always tomorrow."

"I'm glad you agree."

"You didn't get it just now, did you?"

"Didn't you just say that there is always tomorrow?"

"Yes. To show you that you always say "tomorrow"
whenever something is a little more difficult."

"You never give up. Do you?"

"If I give up who will inspire you
to overcome the weakness of doing nothing
while expecting miracles?"

*"All right, but today is Friday,
and you know how I feel on Friday."*

"Friday is the best day to exercise.
We can rest on Sunday.

You'll feel better afterwards."

"I know, but it's still so hard."

"That's just the feeling that comes from being tired.
It'll pass very fast as soon as you begin exercising."

"I hope so."

IV. Hesitator:

"Look at the sunrise. It is so orange
and inviting to welcome the coming day.
I look forward to a cup of coffee and my workout routine."

*"But today is Friday. The day you usually
stay in bed and sleep a little longer."*

"I don't even remember a Friday
I stayed in bed longer than 6 AM.
Come on. It will be a great day."

V. Master:

"Look at this sky. I am so happy I don't sleep.
It's time for a cup of coffee and a workout.
I love Fridays."

BMI (Body Mass Index)

Scenario 2. Jen is 110 pounds. She lost thirty pounds in the last six months, but is weak and constantly tired. According to her BMI (Body Mass Index), she was considered obese before losing weight. Curiously, her body fat percentage classified her as obese after losing weight as well. She wonders how this can be.

I. Fatalist:

*"That's ridiculous.
It's impossible to have a perfect BMI
and still be obese. There must be
something wrong with the measurements."*

II. Disbeliever:

*"That's ridiculous.
It's impossible to have a perfect BMI
and still be obese. There must be
something wrong with measurements."*

"I thought you knew
that BMI is the relationship
between height and weight,
so it cannot measure body fat,
and it cannot show whether

or not someone is obese."

"But my measurements show I had
35 % body fat when I weighed 140 pounds,
and even though I am so much thinner,
I have the same 35 % today.
Don't you see it's illogical?"

"Well, it's definitely a problem,
but I don't see it is a measurement problem."

"Look. BMI is medically proven,
and used in almost every medical office,
so I'd better use it as a point of reference."

III. Debater:

"That's ridiculous.
It's impossible to have a perfect BMI
and still be obese. There must be
something wrong with measurements."

"Don't try to pretend that
you don't know what happened."

"Maybe you can enlighten me,
because I'm completely puzzled by this."

"It's very simple, because all you did

was run on a treadmill, so
you burned muscle instead of fat.
That's why you became weak, and your energy dropped."

"But, then why is my BMI normal,
even though I am obese?"

"Come on. We covered that already.
BMI is misleading.
You should know that by now."

"Have you lost your mind?
Don't you know that BMI
is used by the whole medical community?"

"That's true, but they are mistaken.
We shouldn't be scared to say so.
You have to think for yourself.
BMI stands for Body Mass Index,
but when you calculate it, you enter
your height and body weight,
so it really should be called
Height Weight Index. That's why you can
have a normal BMI and be 'skinny-obese' or 'skinny-lean.'"

"If you are so smart, tell me what I should do?"

"Don't use the BMI. Forget all about it.
Your body fat percentage is

35%, so it qualifies you as obese
though you only weigh110 pounds.
This means you are missing 20 pounds of muscle,
which will take you two years to restore.
You wouldn't know any of this by using the BMI."

"But how could this misleading information be spread so widely?

"Let's not focus on that.
Let's measure the body fat percentage again,
and come up with a plan
to gain back your muscle."

"I'm all for it."

"Great, let's have fun and get better."

IV. Hesitator:

"After a year I am as obese as when I started.
This BMI method can be very inaccurate.
From now on, I will use a body fat measuring device.

"But the whole medical community cannot be mistaken?"

"Maybe they aren't, although
being vague doesn't help anyone.

It's better to know the real numbers.
So, let's recover your muscle and strength."

V. Master:

"I knew there was something wrong with the BMI,
but I couldn't understand what it was.
It's great that I measured my body fat,
otherwise I would be unable to help myself.
It's time to stop running on a treadmill, and build muscle."

HEART

Scenario 3. Jen's cardiologist tells her she needs to run at least 30 minutes a day to keep her heart healthy.

I. Fatalist:

"How many time have I said
that sprinting and yoga
isn't enough exercise
to have a healthy heart?"
It's good that I didn't cancel
my gym membership.
I can run on the treadmill tonight."

II. Disbeliever:

"How many time have I said
that sprinting and yoga
isn't enough exercise
to have a healthy heart?"
It's good that I didn't cancel
my gym membership.
I can run on the treadmill tonight."

"But before you go, you should know
that there are places where people
live more than one hundred years,
and all they do is gardening."

"You must mean Russia,
where people claim to live
until one hundred and twenty,
although nobody can prove it."

"There are books written about
these places. The writers call
them Blue Zones—the villages
where people forget to die."

"Books are great for amusement,
but as soon as you want to apply
their guidelines, you learn
how they can also be deceptive.
Nothing beats the treadmill."

III. Debater:

"How many time have I said
that sprinting and yoga
isn't enough exercise
to have a healthy heart?"
It's good that I didn't cancel
my gym membership.
I can run on the treadmill tonight."

"Doesn't a sprinter have a healthy heart?"

"I know for sure that every time

a doctor is concerned about his patient's heart,
he sends him to run a long distance.
He definitely does not tell the patient to sprint."

"That's because they don't know any better.
All they know is to raise the heart rate,
and the simplest way to do that,
is to have their patients run."

"You always believe that there
is a conspiracy in the world,
that people lie because the truth
is not convenient."

"You must be feeling the truth.
I have never seen you so upset."

"Of course I am.
You can die if you don't listen."

"I can also die while running marathons.
Isn't it what happens during those competitions?"

"Ha! And you say that I am the one who overreacts.
The cardiologist asks for only 30 minutes
of running, not hours."

"I just don't want to exhaust myself.
When I sprint I feel happy and rejuvenated,
and when I watch people running on a treadmill,

it makes me feel kind of sick."

"No pain, no gain. Don't you know that?"

"I don't like pain, or making myself tired.
Let's do double sprints during the week
and test our heart in three months."

"What if the heart gets worse?"

"Then I will run on the treadmill."

*"I look forward to seeing
you disappointed."*

IV. Hesitator:

"This doctor doesn't know how
damaging long distance
running can be to a heart."

*"How can you say such a thing?
He's not just any doctor.
He's a cardiologist."*

"There are many cardiologists
who have bad hearts only because
they live the wrong way.
I will not follow them."

V. Master

"Sprinters don't die while running,
and some of them still run
with their own joints and healthy hearts,
even when they are over one hundred.
Time to run some sprints."

CALORIES

Scenario 4. Jen wants to lose weight but she does not want to agree to eat less, so if she wants to lose one pound of fat a week, she needs to run for at least two hours everyday.

I. Fatalist:

"That's fantastic. I can eat
just as before and lose all that fat.
Nothing could be better.
I will start in the morning."

II. Disbeliever:

"That's fantastic. I can eat
just as before and lose all that fat.
Nothing could be better.
I will start in the morning."

"But you have never exercised before,
and running for two hours is extreme.
Shouldn't you compromise?
What about eating
and exercising less?"

"I don't want to eat less.
Food is sacred to me,

so eating less would be mortifying."

"I just cannot imagine how
you will find the time.
You already sleep only 5 hours."

"That's easy.
I'll do my work
while running."

III. Debater:

"That's fantastic. I can eat
just as before and lose all that fat.
Nothing could be better.
I will start in the morning."

"I knew you were crazy,
but this beats all your previous ideas.
Why do you fuss so much about eating a little less?
All this running will equal only half of a bagel in calories.
I think the real reason is to have an excuse
to quit when you get sore and tired."

"It's only two hours.
I'm sure I can do it for three months."

"And, then what?"

"What do you mean 'what'?
I will simply enjoy my skinny jeans."

"Will you still run?"

"Of course not, silly.
I'll be resting after all this running."

"But then you will get fat
just as fast as you got skinny."

"No, I won't. I know how to maintain my weight."

"Well, as you know, as soon as you stop
running you will eat more than you need,
like you always have,
and a half bagel everyday
will end up as fat."

"So I will eat less."

"Why not eat less from the beginning,
so you get used to it while getting ready for those jeans?"

"I just hate eating less."

"But we both know that it is crucial,
so if you really want to succeed,
just start with eating less dense foods,
so the volume will stay the same
but you'll take in fewer calories."

"That can't be true."

"It is. Do you want to try it?"

"Why not."

IV. Hesitator:

"Running for two hours everyday
can't be good for anybody.
What If I eat less?"

*"But running is a cardiovascular exercise
and your cardiologist told you that you need it anyway."*

"You're right.
But I can do cardiovascular training
without running at all."

"It's impossible."

"No, it isn't impossible at all.
Do ten squats and your
heart will pump fast.
And it will not stop
even when you sit on a bench to rest.
Let's do some sets of squats."

V. Master:

"I am happy knowing that
I don't have to run to lose weight.
Tonight, for one week,
I will start keeping a food journal.
Then, I will calculate how many fewer calories
I need to lose one pound a week.
It's a good feeling to know this can be done."

STRENGTH

Scenario 5. Jen looks at her progress chart, and sees that she did not gain any strength in the last half year.

I. Fatalist:

"This program obviously doesn't work for me.
Maybe it works for somebody else,
but there must be something wrong with it
since my body is not improving.
It's time to find a different program."

II. Disbeliever:

"This program obviously doesn't work for me.
Maybe it works for somebody else,
but there must be something wrong with it
since my body is not improving.
It's time to find a different program."

"How can a program not work?
It was designed to make you stronger.
What is wrong with it?"

"Maybe the creator was a wishful thinker.
How can the same program work for everyone?

"Did you really give it a chance,
and follow it all the way through?"

"I used it for three months.
Isn't that enough time to get results?
I'm sure you will like this new program.
It was created by an athlete,
and people who use it swear that it works.
We'll start tomorrow.
You will love it."

III. Debater:

"This program obviously doesn't work for me.
Maybe it works for somebody else,
but there must be something wrong with it
since my body is not improving.
It's time to find a different program."

"But you didn't follow the program one hundred percent.
And the last time you failed,
you said the same thing.
Isn't it time to look yourself straight
in the eye and admit you got bored."

"That's exactly why I couldn't succeed.
It's boring."

"How can a program be boring?"

"What kind of question is that?
You do the same thing everyday,
and after a while it becomes boring.
Isn't that normal?"

"Programs don't make people feel things.
We're responsible for our own feelings."

"Come on, you know what I mean."

"No, I don't. Tell me."

"I like to have fun and enjoy
new things. It makes me feel alive."

"Think about all those athletes
who do the same thing over and over
and never get bored.
If doing the same is always boring,
then you would have to say that
swimming is boring,
and you know that it's not."

"That's logical, but life is often full of surprises.
For example, when I go to a gym
and see all the people on treadmills

watching the news and being relaxed,
I forget all about getting stronger.
All I think about is getting on a treadmill
and moving like everyone else."

"What if you keep a training log
so you know how much stronger you become?

"Sure, but what if it doesn't work?"

"It will work if you follow the program
without looking for excuses."

"I'm just disappointed, that's all."

"Just give me three months to show you,
and I'm sure you will like it too."

"Three months?"

"Yes."

"Okay. But if it doesn't work,
we'll find something new that works."

"Sure."

IV. Hesitator:

"I must have been doing something wrong.
My strength didn't improve at all even though
I train twice a day. I have to ask
a weightlifting coach to help me."

"You don't need any help.
Getting stronger is not a fast process.
Just keep doing what you are doing."

"I know it, although no change
after all those months tells me
that something is not quite right.
I will call a coach tomorrow."

V. Master:

"Trying on my own is not working.
Getting stronger is not my expertise.
Tomorrow, I'll meet a weightlifting coach."

BULKY

Scenario 6. A friend tells Jen to stop weightlifting because she could become bulky.

I. Fatalist:

"Terrible! I didn't know
I could look like a man
simply by lifting weights,
although I remember this Russian
weightlifter who weighed almost 400 pounds.
I'd better stop now, so I won't be sorry
when I look like a man."

II. Disbeliever:

"Terrible! I didn't know
I could look like a man
by simply lifting weights.
although I remember this Russian,
weightlifter who weighed almost 400 pounds.
I'd better stop now so I won't be sorry
when I look like a man."

"Isn't that an exaggeration?
You probably would need to lift
a lot of weights to grow muscles

the size of a man's. But, if you did,
it should be easy to lose the muscle
if you don't want it anymore."

"*It isn't so simple.*
I've seen many bodybuilders stuck
with their bulky bodies forever."

"But you are not a bodybuilder,
you are just an ordinary woman
who wants to be fit and healthy,
and weightlifting helps."

"*I always thought that it was weird*
for a woman to lift weights.
And now others say it, too.
I've never liked it anyway.
No more struggling with weights.
It's time for fun.
Nothing could be better than running
on a treadmill while watching a movie."

III. Debater:

"*Terrible! I didn't know*
I could look like a man
by simply lifting weights,
although I remember this Russian
weightlifter who weighed almost 400 pounds.

*I'd better stop now so I won't be sorry
when I look like a man."*

"I don't think you should worry about
becoming bulky. Have you forgotten
that when we age we lose muscle?
You couldn't become bulky even if you wanted to."

*"You probably read new age magazines
telling you all these lies so you'll go to a gym
and recover the precious muscle you lost while aging.
Advertisements are designed to scare
baby boomers so they go to gyms and hire trainers."*

"What about just observing life?
Don't you see that most old people become skinny,
stooped-over and weak, and if they are big
they carry mostly fat on their brittle bones
with little muscle left?"

*"You must have special goggles
to look inside a body."*

"No. Just a caliper to measure body fat."

*"And of course you've measured everyone
you pass on a street."*

"I don't have to measure them,
I know from the research,

and I can see."

"I'm sorry you still trust researchers.
Don't you know that these days you can order
any research and any outcome you desire?"

"That's your world. No trust.
But this only helps you fail
whenever you like.
Don't you care?

"It's you who doesn't care
about being bulky."

"I just know it isn't possible."

"What if it is?"

"Then I will apologize."

"That will be fun."

"Let's do the measurements and check in a month."

"Fantastic."

IV. Hesitator:

"I guess he doesn't know
that it's not easy to be bulky.
Athletes train for years to achieve it."

*"But maybe your genetics
are prone to muscle growth?"*

"Genetics? Have you lost your mind?
Let's not waste time, and go to the gym
to lift some weights instead.
Muscle doesn't grow
while resting, fat does."

V. Master:

"No wonder people become weak.
Where is a weightlifting gym?"

SWEAT

Scenario 7. Jen's friend tells her she needs to sweat to get the benefit of exercise.

I. Fatalist:

"To sweat is life.
But you are never tired; you only sprint,
lift heavy weights, and stretch.
Finally, a true friend tells you
that sweating is necessary to be healthy.
I look forward to exercising harder,
and feeling the sweat rolling down my skin."

II. Disbeliever:

"To sweat is life.
But you are never tired; you only sprint,
lift heavy weights, and stretch.
Finally, a true friend tells you
that sweating is necessary to be healthy.
I look forward to exercising harder,
and feeling the sweat rolling down my skin."

"I thought that the purpose of exercise
is to get stronger and flexible, not just to sweat.

What if all this exercise madness is just about
selling athletic shoes and food bars?"

"If it was, then millions of people
wouldn't search for new and better
routines to make them sweat."

"That's exactly what I said.
They look for a way to sweat, not for strength."

"What are you talking about?"

"Sweat means strength.
This is clearly accepted
by all the best athletes.
So, let's follow the winners."

"Winners sweat.
Losers watch.
Let's break some sweat."

III. Debater:

"To sweat is life.
But you are never tired; you only sprint,
lift heavy weights, and stretch.
Finally, a true friend tells you
that sweating is necessary to be healthy.
I look forward to exercising harder,

and feeling the sweat rolling down my skin."

"Don't you feel strong, healthy, and happy?

*"Yes, I do. That's why I want to push
even harder; to get stronger."*

"But you should know that as soon as
you sweat, you have exercised too much.
The body cannot recover anymore,
so it gets weaker, slows down,
and becomes less powerful.
The best way to exercise is to be efficient."

*"I cannot think of a better way
of training for efficiency
than to train hard and sweat a lot.
But, maybe you know, so enlighten me."*

"Well, it is very simple.
If you run the same distance faster,
you become more efficient."

*"So could you say that the more
you sweat in the same amount of time,
the more efficient you become?"*

"Sure, but...."

*"I heard the word 'but.' But, isn't
that always the case with you?
Whenever I'm right you say, 'but.'"*

"It's different this time."

"Tell me how."

"It's true that the more you sweat,
the more efficient you become.
But, when a runner's body sweats,
it becomes hot and inflamed,
and it cannot sustain the speed,
so it naturally slows down
and become less efficient."

*"Are you sure about that?
Is there any proof?"*

"Of course, there is, but
just simple logic is enough.
Isn't it?"

*"It seems so but I have to check
with a scientist, anyway."*

"Of course."

IV. Hesitator:

"I don't get why people
don't see that the most powerful
athletes don't sweat at all.
I'm taking about sprinters, gymnasts,
pole-vaulters, just to mention a few."

*"But many athletes sweat, for example
basketball and football players
sweat a lot, just to name a few."*

"Yes, they sweat, but mostly
because of enduring the competition
of the game. They don't sweat
while training for power, and
we need more power to handle
all the physical challenges in life.
So, let's not add sweat to our training
and become powerless."

V. Master:

"It's amazing that people compromise
quality for quantity, while everyone knows
that nothing feels better than being powerful.
Sweat destroys quality.
Let's keep that in mind."

MUSCLE CONFUSION

Scenario 8. Jen is reading a book that says she needs to change her exercises every day, to confuse the muscles so they will grow.

I. Fatalist:

"I always hated doing the same exercise over and over.
Now, science finally proves it is not only wrong,
it can actually stop my progress.
From today on, there will be a lot of confusion."

II. Disbeliever:

"I always hated doing the same exercise over and over.
Now finally the science proves it is not only wrong
it can actually stop my progress.
From today on there will be a lot of confusion."

"Shouldn't you spend a certain amount of time
practicing the same routine
for months to improve your skills?"

"If you do, you get bored
and stop striving for more.
It's wonderful that science supports this,
so I don't have to spend

a lot of time convincing you.”

"I thought that by practicing
over and over we surpass difficulty,
get better and want to practice even harder."

*"It's great that you don't decide
how we exercise, otherwise
we would suffer like rats in a trap."*

III. Debater:

*"I always hated doing the same exercise over and over.
Now finally the science proves it is not only wrong
it can actually stop my progress.
From today on there will be a lot of confusion."*

"Have you ever seen a confused pianist?"

*"Piano is about becoming more skillful,
not about getting stronger and building bigger muscles."*

"What about a gymnast or a weightlifter?
Don't they practice their routine to perfection?
And, aren't they the strongest of all athletes?"

*"They will never tell you what they do.
It is a top secret so they can win the Olympics.
There is a lot of confusion about how to train."*

"I thought that people want to
do a different routine every day
simply because they are bored."

*"Well, it's no fun to keep
doing the same thing, is it?"*

"Have you ever seen a bored gymnast?"

"There are many of them in gyms."

"And what does the coach say to them?"

"I don't know. Tell me."

"Find yourself a beam."

"A beam? What does that mean?"

"Come on. Use your imagination."

*"Something different, I guess, to stimulate them.
That would prove the whole muscle confusion theory."*

"Ha! I thought you might conclude that.
But it really means that if you don't
pay attention to what you're doing
you will fall and hurt yourself."

"So you propose fear as the answer?"

"No, not fear. Difficulty.
By making what is difficult easy,
we becoming better
at anything we practice.
That's the best way to progress.
Stay focused, not confused."

"Even though you are bored?"

"Boredom changes when we progress
and see greatness just over the horizon.
Give me three months and I will show you
the joy of repeating the same routine."

*"I can survive for three months.
But if I'm bored after that,
we will try muscle confusion.
Okay?"*

"Okay."

IV. Hesitator:

"It's amazing what people can do
to deal with their boredom.

They will entertain themselves, even though
it means no progress anymore."

"I wouldn't be so sure.
I see some value in being entertained."

"Yes, there is some value.
There is nothing wrong with it.
But, it's not the exercise that's boring; it's the people.
Let's accept what we did yesterday, and make it better today."

V. Master:

"I'm glad formula one drivers don't buy into muscle confusion.
It would be painful to see a confused driver.
If making something perfect is a pleasure,
then becoming perfect is pure music.
Let's play some for the world."

READING A BILLBOARD

Scenario 9. As Jen drives on a freeway, a billboard with an ad captures her attention:

"With this new proven exercise program
you will gain 63 pounds of muscle
in only 28 days."

I. Fatalist:

"Wow! That's incredible.
Finally, science is freeing us from atrophy.
I only need to gain 15 pounds of muscle,
so it shouldn't take me longer than a week.
I love this."

II. Disbeliever:

"Wow! That's incredible.
Finally, science is freeing us from atrophy.
I only need to gain 15 pounds of muscle,
so it shouldn't take me longer than a week.
I love this."

"That's a lot of muscle to gain.
Don't you think this ad
is a bit of an exaggeration?"

"Well, it means only one thing:
The old world is changing,
and finally, I can gain back
the lost muscle in no time.
What a wonderful time to be alive."

"But it means you would gain
more than two pounds a week."

"I know. It's awesome!
I'm buying it right now."

III. Debater:

"Wow! That's incredible.
Finally, science is freeing us from atrophy.
I only need to gain 15 pounds of muscle,
so it shouldn't take me longer than a week.
I love this."

"And, of course you don't see anything wrong with it?"

"Wrong?
You must be talking about yourself.
You're the one who always finds something wrong.
So tell me, what's wrong now?"

"It's physically impossible, that's what's wrong.

And even if it was possible, you would need to
consume about 2000 more calories a day
just to build that muscle."

"*That's even better.*
Eating more to build muscle—
what could be better than that?"

"Apparently, you didn't hear me.
There isn't an athlete on this planet
who has actually done that.
It's not even close."

"*Why do we talk about athletes?*
This is a new scientific breakthrough.
Athletes will learn from it."

"Come on. Even animals don't grow so fast.
It takes four years for a cow to grow into
a thousand pound adult.
That's not even a pound a day.
You're talking about two pounds."

"*We aren't animals.*
We have science."

"Okay, tell you what.
If we ask any trainer and he agrees

that growing more than two pounds of muscle
a day is possible, we'll buy the program and test it."

"Sounds good."

IV. Hesitator:

"How could anyone believe such a thing?
Let's just go to the gym and lift some weights."

"But, what if it is possible?
You could gain all these pounds in a flash."

"It's definitely tempting,
although I'm too logical and too old
to jump on an insane offer."

"You never know."

"This I know."

V. Master:

"If I was desperate, or I didn't know better,
I could lose both money and time.
But I do know, so I'll spend them

going to the gym for a year
to grow all this muscle,
And I think there will even be enough
to have a weightlifting session with a coach.
I feel so fortunate to know what is real."

WATCHING TV

Scenario 10. Jen is lying on the couch watching her favorite TV show. As she reaches for another walnut, a commercial pops out:

"In only 8 minutes of exercise a day, you will not only lose all the weight you want to shed, but you will look younger and more attractive."

I. Fatalist:

"Poor people, they still believe
they need to exercise.
What could be better than
lying on a couch and eating nuts
one by one, chewing and swallowing
until you are full?"

II. Disbeliever:

"Poor people, they still believe
they need to exercise.
What could be better than
lying on a couch and eating nuts
one by one, chewing and swallowing
until you are full?"

"But you're more than 300 pounds
and your doctor says you are pre-diabetic."

"Oh, she's just like all the others,
she bought into the lie."

"It's not a lie. You are sick
and you can die at any time."

"Oh, shut up. You're like the others, too.
Scared of your own shadow."

III. Debater:

"Poor people, they still believe
they need to exercise.
What could be better than
lying on a couch and eating nuts
one by one, chewing and swallowing
until you are full?"

"You must be completely lost.
Don't you see how sick you've become?
Your blood pressure is up,
your cholesterol is high,
you take more than five different medications,
and, worst of all, you can't find a friend."

"As usual you exaggerate. Look around.
Almost everyone is big and takes medication.
It's the normal way. You don't want me
to run like a rat on a treadmill, do you?"

"It's not only about that.
I want you to be healthy
and live a long, long time."

"Don't worry. I will. And if not, that's life."

"It's always the same story with you."

"Is there any other story?"

"What if there is a way to be
more youthful and happier?"

"I would be the first one to know it."

"But how can you know it without trying it?
We could start with this program
It's really good."

"You really believe that it's real?"

"Yes, I do."

"Well, I guess we could try it,
but only for a month."

"Wonderful."

IV. Hesitator:

"It sounds good. I should probably buy it."

"But then you'll be running like a rat
on a treadmill, and miss
watching movies in the evening.
You know how much you love to watch them."

"But it's only 8 minutes a day."

"Come on. You know it's not true. They lie
so you will buy their program, and then
eight minutes becomes two hours everyday."

"You're right, although I know
that not all of them are liars.
I'll try it for a month and see
if I lose any weight and feel better."

V. Master:

"It's good to know that weight loss
has nothing to do with exercise.
But the exercise routine can help me
get stronger and regain my muscle.
I'll order the program and try it."

MARATHON

Scenario 11. Jen is talking to a friend who invites her to prepare to run a marathon.

I. Fatalist:

"Wow! Running a marathon.
I never thought I could
endure such an incredible challenge.
Nothing in my life comes close
to matching such heights.
I will join the team tomorrow morning
on the five mile run, and begin
my journey to become superhuman."

II. Disbeliever:

"Wow! Running a marathon.
I never thought I could
endure such an incredible challenge.
Nothing in my life comes close
to matching such heights.
I will join the team tomorrow morning
on the five mile run, and begin
my journey to become superhuman."

"I've read that sometimes during a race
as many as three marathoners die,
and others end up in hospitals
because of dehydration and exhaustion.
Don't you think that attempting
such a strenuous sport is too risky?
We can always run sprints to become faster."

"Where did you get such a fatalistic attitude?
There are millions of marathon runners, and
it's quite normal that accidents happen."

"Three people dying in a race is
not an accident and, by the way,
sprinters don't just die while running.
There are millions of sprinters out there."

"I think you're just lazy,
and you will say anything to keep me
from even attempting to run a marathon.
Get ready because tomorrow we will act like champions.
You'll love it when we win."

III. Debater:

"Wow! Running a marathon.
I never thought I could
endure such an incredible challenge.
Nothing in my life comes close

to matching such heights.
I will join the team tomorrow morning
on the five mile run, and begin
my journey to become superhuman."

"Why on Earth would you run a marathon?
Don't you know that it is about survival?
Marathoners stress their organs to the max,
so the body can keep running
even while breaking apart."

"Every athlete stresses the body to the max.
It's the nature of sport."

"All I know is that endurance athletes
constantly complain about being tired and in pain,
and power athletes never do."

"Power athletes? What are you talking about?
Marathoners are power athletes, too."

"Come on, you know that power means
running fast, not running until you drop dead."

"Look everyone knows that marathon
runners are the most powerful."

"Well, it's easy to test. Power
simply means distance covered divided by time.
So, the faster you run the same distance,

the more powerful you are.
Or, the further you run in the same
amount of time, the more powerful you are.

*"But, a marathon runner runs for two hours.
A sprinter could never keep up."*

"That's true, although a sprinter runs
10 meters in one second while a marathon runner
takes two seconds. So the sprinter is twice as
powerful as the marathon runner."

"It can't be true. I'll have to test it."

"Sorry to disillusion you."

"Hey, you haven't, yet."

"Okay, let's wait until you get the results."

IV. Hesitator:

"I don't think it's a good idea.
It will take too much time and effort,
and cause too much pain."

*"If you work with a coach,
it doesn't have to be painful."*

"Sure. Although I don't have two or three
hours a day to prove that I am great.
I can do it on a track."

V. Master:

"I will not expose my body to this
kind of exhaustion and stress,
but I used to run, and I miss it,
so I will do some sprints tomorrow."

TRAINER

Scenario 12. Jen is talking to a trainer who just told her that she needs to run on a treadmill for two hours every day to lose an excess of thirty pounds of fat, and gain 20 pounds of muscle.

I. Fatalist:

*"That's great. I like that this trainer is tough.
I'll lose this fat in no time."*

II. Disbeliever:

*"That's great. I like that this trainer is tough.
I'll lose this fat in no time."*

"But doesn't that also mean you'll lose muscle?
He told you that you have to gain twenty pounds of it
and that it will take you at least two years."

*"Let's not worry about that. He knows what he's doing.
After all, he is a personal trainer and we pay
for his professional advice and assistance."*

"It's just that I cannot imagine how you can build muscle
by doing exercises that burn muscle."

"I told you already. Stop worrying.
Have faith in the trainer.
He would never do what
isn't scientifically proven."

III. Debater:

"That's great. I like that this trainer is tough.
I'll lose this fat in no time."

"Of course it will be fast.
You will burn lots of muscle, stay fat,
get thin, weak, tired and start eating more.
Haven't you already gone down that road many times?"

"This time is different. Look at this trainer.
He is lean and handsome. He definitely knows
how to help other people to become what he is."

"He is also twenty years old, while you're fifty."

"So should I learn from a sixty year old
who has a belly, wears old clothes,
and complains about his body?"

"Be serious. What can you learn from
a twenty year old—partying all night?
Always looking into a mirror?"

*"There are young people who are not
only about rock and roll and a mirror."*

"That's true, although twenty year olds
don't need to train in a gym.
They are in school learning
from old people how the body ages."

"But I'm not inspired by old people."

"Would you be inspired by a trainer
older than you who is as strong as
a twenty year old and as wise as a sage?"

"Of course I would, but it's not possible to find one."

"It is, and I will find you that trainer."

"Okay, but if you don't, we stay with this one."

"Alright."

IV. Hesitator:

"This trainer is too young to learn from.
I'd better find somebody who
knows from experience how to help
an already aged body."

"But look at him, he is so handsome.
Can you imagine working out
every day and being spotted by him?"

"I can imagine how wonderful I would feel
and how everyone in the gym would be jealous,
but I also can imagine how he would
make us run on the treadmill
while he admires himself in the mirror.
We would lose muscle, get weaker
and become older even more quickly than we do now.
So, let's stop dreaming, and find somebody
who can actually help."

V. Master:

"I know that it's easy to break
an already aging body,

but it's very difficult to heal it.
So, let's say thank you for the great
amusement, and find somebody
who is old enough to help us work
with the body that we have."

Part II
Practice Personalizing the Book's 12 Scenarios

What Would the Master within Me Say?
What Would the Fatalist within Me Say?

Make the Master's voice the last in the Debate.

WAKING UP

Scenario 1. You are sleeping. It is 6 AM and the alarm just went off to remind you to go to the gym and workout.

Fatalist:

F _____

Disbeliever:

F _____

M_____

F _____

Debater:

F _____

M_____

F _____

M_____

F _____

M_____

Hesitator:

F _____

M_____

F _____

Master:

F _____

BMI (Body Mass Index)

Scenario 2. You are 110 pounds. You lost thirty pounds in the last six months, but you are weak and constantly tired. According to your BMI (Body Mass Index), you were considered obese before losing weight. Curiously, your body fat percentage classified you as obese after losing weight as well. You wonder how this can be.

Fatalist:

F _____

Disbeliever:

F _____

M_____

F _____

Debater:

F _____

M_____

F _____

M_____

F _____

M_____

Hesitator:

F _____

M_____

F _____

Master:

F _____

HEART

Scenario 3. Your cardiologist tells you that you need to run at least 30 minutes a day to keep your heart healthy.

Fatalist:

F _____

Disbeliever:

F _____

M_____

F _____

Debater:

F _____

M_____

F _____

M_____

F _____

M_____

Hesitator:

F _____

M_____

F _____

Master:

F _____

CALORIES

Scenario 4. You want to lose weight but you do not want to agree to eat less, so if you want to lose one pound of fat a week, you need to run for at least two hours everyday.

Fatalist:

F _____

Disbeliever:

F _____

M_____

F _____

Debater:

F _____

M_____

F _____

M_____

F _____

M_____

Hesitator:

F _____

M_____

F _____

Master:

F _____

STRENGTH

Scenario 5. You look at your progress chart, and see that you did not gain any strength in the last half year.

Fatalist:

F _____

Disbeliever:

F _____

M_____

F _____

Debater:

F _____

M_____

F _____

M_____

F _____

M_____

Hesitator:

F _____

M_____

F _____

Master:

F _____

BULKY

Scenario 6. A friend tells you to stop weightlifting because you could become bulky.

Fatalist:

F _____

Disbeliever:

F _____

M_____

F _____

Debater:

F _____

M_____

F _____

M_____

F _____

M_____

Hesitator:

F _____

M_____

F _____

Master:

F _____

SWEAT

Scenario 7. Your friend tells you that you need to sweat to get the benefit of exercise.

Fatalist:

F _____

Disbeliever:

F _____

M_____

F _____

Debater:

F _____

M_____

F _____

M_____

F _____

M_____

Hesitator:

F _____

M_____

F _____

Master:

F _____

MUSCLE CONFUSION

Scenario 8. You are reading a book that says you need to change your exercises every day, to confuse the muscles so they will grow.

Fatalist:
F _____

Disbeliever:
F _____
M_____
F _____

Debater:
F _____
M_____
F _____
M_____
F _____
M_____

Hesitator:
F _____
M_____
F _____

Master:
F _____

READING A BILLBOARD

Scenario 9. As you drive on a freeway, a billboard with an ad captures your attention:

"With this new proven exercise program
you will gain 63 pounds of muscle
in only 28 days."

Fatalist:

F _____

Disbeliever:

F _____

M_____

F _____

Debater:

F _____

M_____

F _____

M_____

F _____

M_____

Hesitator:

F _____

M_____

F _____

Master:

F _____

Scenario 10. You are lying on the couch watching your favorite TV show. As you reach for another walnut, a commercial pops out:

"In only 8 minutes of exercise a day, you will not only lose all the weight you want to shed, but you will look younger and more attractive."

Fatalist:

F _____

Disbeliever:

F _____

M_____

F _____

Debater:

F _____

M_____

F _____

M_____

F _____

M_____

Hesitator:

F _____

M_____

F _____

Master:

F _____

MARATHON

Scenario 11. You are talking to a friend who invites you to prepare to run a marathon.

Fatalist:

F _____

Disbeliever:

F _____

M_____

F _____

Debater:

F _____

M_____

F _____

M_____

F _____

M_____

Hesitator:

F _____

M_____

F _____

Master:

F _____

TRAINER

Scenario 12. You are talking to a trainer who just told you that you need to run on a treadmill for two hours every day to lose an excess of thirty pounds of fat, and gain 20 pounds of muscle.

Fatalist:

F _____

Disbeliever:

F _____

M_____

F _____

Debater:

F _____

M_____

F _____

M_____

F _____

M_____

Hesitator:

F _____

M_____

F _____

Master:

F _____

Part III
Practice Writing Your Own Scenarios

Before writing out the dialogues, describe the basic nature of the situation.

Scenario _____

_____

_____

Fatalist:

F _____

Disbeliever:

F _____

M_____

F _____

Debater:

F _____

M_____

F _____

M_____

F _____

M_____

Hesitator:

F _____

M_____

F _____

Master:

F _____

Scenario _____

_____

_____

Fatalist:

F _____

Disbeliever:

F _____

M_____

F _____

Debater:

F _____

M_____

F _____

M_____

F _____

M_____

Hesitator:

F _____

M_____

F _____

Master:

F _____

Scenario _____

_____

_____

Fatalist:

F _____

Disbeliever:

F _____

M_____

F _____

Debater:

F _____

M_____

F _____

M_____

F _____

M_____

Hesitator:

F _____

M_____

F _____

Master:

F _____

Scenario _____
_____
_____

Fatalist:
F _____

Disbeliever:
F _____
M_____
F _____

Debater:
F _____
M_____
F _____
M_____
F _____
M_____

Hesitator:
F _____
M_____
F _____

Master:
F _____

Scenario _____

_____

_____

Fatalist:

F _____

Disbeliever:

F _____

M_____

F _____

Debater:

F _____

M_____

F _____

M_____

F _____

M_____

Hesitator:

F _____

M_____

F _____

Master:

F _____

Scenario _____

_____

_____

Fatalist:

F _____

Disbeliever:

F _____

M_____

F _____

Debater:

F _____

M_____

F _____

M_____

F _____

M_____

Hesitator:

F _____

M_____

F _____

Master:

F _____

Scenario _____

_____

_____

Fatalist:

F _____

Disbeliever:

F _____

M_____

F _____

Debater:

F _____

M_____

F _____

M_____

F _____

M_____

Hesitator:

F _____

M_____

F _____

Master:

F _____

Scenario _____
_____
_____

Fatalist:
F _____

Disbeliever:
F _____
M_____
F _____

Debater:
F _____
M_____
F _____
M_____
F _____
M_____

Hesitator:
F _____
M_____
F _____

Master:
F _____

Scenario _____

_____

_____

Fatalist:

F _____

Disbeliever:

F _____

M_____

F _____

Debater:

F _____

M_____

F _____

M_____

F _____

M_____

Hesitator:

F _____

M_____

F _____

Master:

F _____

Scenario _____

_____

_____

Fatalist:

F _____

Disbeliever:

F _____

M_____

F _____

Debater:

F _____

M_____

F _____

M_____

F _____

M_____

Hesitator:

F _____

M_____

F _____

Master:

F _____

Scenario _____

_____

_____

Fatalist:

F _____

Disbeliever:

F _____

M_____

F _____

Debater:

F _____

M_____

F _____

M_____

F _____

M_____

Hesitator:

F _____

M_____

F _____

Master:

F _____

Scenario _____

_____

_____

Fatalist:

F _____

Disbeliever:

F _____

M_____

F _____

Debater:

F _____

M_____

F _____

M_____

F _____

M_____

Hesitator:

F _____

M_____

F _____

Master:

F _____

Please don't be discouraged if you fail in any situation. Begin by clearly identifying it. Then write out the five-level dialogue, using the formula provided in the templates above. Pinpoint the level at which you currently find yourself. Practice "importing" the message from level five into your real-life scenario (self conditioning), until the voice of the Master within you triumphs.

For information on *The Happy Body* Program, including possible updates relating to The Way of Conscious Eating, please visit TheHappyBody.com.

You are always welcome to share your personal success story with the author, via Jerzy@TheHappyBody.com.

Choose the arts; they become your emotions.
Choose your emotions; they become your feelings.
Choose your feelings; they become your images.
Choose your images; they become your words.
Choose you words; they become your thoughts.

—Jerzy Gregorek

Watch your thoughts; they become words.
Watch your words; they become actions.
Watch your actions; they become habit.
Watch your habits; they become character.
Watch your character; it becomes your destiny.

—Lao Tzu

CONTRARY CONVICTIONS	
The Fatalist	**The Master**
It's too hard.	I know it's hard but I want the benefits.
It's impossible.	It's possible.
I love food too much to eat less.	I love good health enough to eat less.
I'm too old to change.	It's never too late to change.
It's not normal at my age to be thin.	Being trim at any age is healthier.
I'm already old.	I can become more youthful.
I'll die if I eat so little.	Eating appropriately will extend my life.
I won't get enough nutrition.	I eat only nutritious food.
I still don't believe it's possible.	I'll try it and see.

I would starve myself.	If I lose too much weight, I can eat more.
I'm heavier because I'm on my period.	My period is no excuse for gaining weight.
It's not fun to always control oneself.	I can have fun while controlling myself.
Only poor people cook these days.	Intelligent people cook for themselves.
Being fat is normal.	Being trim is normal for healthy people.
Life is short, so enjoy it while you can.	I refuse to shorten my life.
I don't trust science.	I acknowledge reality.
I trust my appetite.	I trust my knowledge.
I don't care about others.	My actions take others into account.
I'll party until I drop.	I'll have fun in a way that's good for me.
I can't get by eating so little.	I will eat only as much as I need to.
I won't struggle with what's difficult.	I won't avoid what's difficult.
I've hit a plateau.	I plan my plateaus.
Nothing works.	Everything works.
I love to get things for free.	I prefer to earn what I get.
Protecting my health is a waste of time.	Protecting my health saves time.
Constant planning is annoying.	Planning is liberating.
I'll do it tomorrow.	I'll do it today.
I hate the clock.	The clock is my friend.
I don't like to do boring things.	Anything can be interesting.
I prefer to live in a fantasy.	I prefer to have both feet on the ground.
People irritate me.	People help me give meaning to my life.
I need more.	I only need enough.
I can't lose weight no matter what I do.	There are many options for losing weight.
I live for the moment.	I live for the long term.
I wish I could buy fitness.	I'm happy I can achieve fitness for myself.
Getting older is depressing.	Life can be enjoyable at any age.
"Enough" is never enough.	"Enough" is always enough.

I'll stop eating when I feel satisfied.	I'll stop eating when I've had enough.
I'll be happy to have finished my work.	I'm happy to be working.
I don't believe in criticizing my friends.	A true friend is always honest.
I want others to inspire me.	I love to inspire myself.
Diets don't work.	Every diet works.
I complain when something is wrong.	I fix what is wrong.
I hope I'll eat less.	I will eat less.
I offer advice to anyone about anything.	I only advise in my area of expertise.
Eating is everything.	Living is everything.
I wish my excess fat would disappear.	I'm responsible for reducing my excess fat.
I blame food companies for my obesity.	I tune out unhealthy advertising.
I fear being hungry.	I fear overeating.
Packaged foods are the most appealing.	Fresh produce is the best kind of food.
I'm not interested in how foods are made.	I want to know how my food is produced.
I want a pill to suppress my appetite.	I decide what goes in my mouth and when.
I'm not smart enough.	I have what it takes.
I could never be like that.	I can be whatever I want to be.
I don't deserve that.	I am as worthy as anyone else is.
"Life is short: eat dessert first."	Life is long: eat healthy food first.
I don't have time.	I always have time for what's important.
I don't have the energy for change.	I'll get stronger, so I'll have more energy.
I was born this way.	I focus on becoming better.
I can't fight my genes.	I can fit into my jeans.
Actors and models are paid to be thin.	Being fit and trim will increase my options.
You can't fight destiny.	I create my own destiny.
"The devil made me do it."	I can be my own angel.
I can't change my environment.	I choose how I respond to my environment.
WRITE YOUR OWN PAIRS	

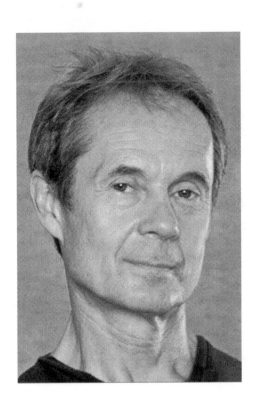

ABOUT THE AUTHOR

Jerzy Gregorek immigrated to the United States together with his wife, Aniela, from Poland in 1986, as political refugees during the Solidarity Movement. An accomplished athlete, he subsequently won four World Weightlifting Championships and established one world record. In 2000, Jerzy and Aniela founded UCLA's weightlifting team, becoming its head coaches. As co-creator of *The Happy Body* Program, Jerzy has been mentoring people for more than 30 years, helping them attain a happy and healthy lifestyle.

In 1998, Jerzy earned an MFA in writing from the Vermont College of Fine Arts. His poems and translations have appeared in numerous publications, including *The American Poetry Review*. His poem "Family Tree" was the winner of *Amelia* magazine's Charles William Duke Longpoem Award in 1998.

In 2002, the National Endowment for the Arts awarded Jerzy a literature fellowship to support the translation from Polish into English of selected poems by Maurycy Szymel. This culminated in the publication in 2013 of *The Shy Hand of a Jew* by Cross-Cultural Communications, which the following year published a collection of Jerzy's own poetry, entitled *Sacred and Scared*. *A Healthy Mirror for Change: Nourishing an Appetite for Losing Weight*, another volume of poetry, was also published in 2014.

This latest book harnesses the power of the discovery of a series of internal dialogues, to help readers achieve important goals in the realm of health and fitness. This is accomplished first by understanding the tension and interplay between the voices of what are termed the Fatalist and the Master within all of us. Readers are then invited to first extend these dialogues into their own lives—and subsequently to articulate other key scenarios in their lives that are playing themselves out along similar lines. Ultimately, by importing the critical message into these various scenarios, you enable the voice of the Master within you to triumph.

Jerzy lives with his wife and their daughter in Woodside, California.

Printed in Great Britain
by Amazon